UNDERSTANDING WOMEN'S GUT HEALTH

EXPLORING THE MICROBIOME-BRAIN CONNECTION
TO MANAGE IBS, SIBO & OTHER DIGESTIVE
DISORDERS THROUGH THE POWER OF FOOD &
NATURAL ALTERNATIVES

JULIA MORENO

CONTENTS

INTRODUCTION

Have you experienced digestive issues? I know I have. I've suffered from bloating, gas, and constipation for many years.

These digestive symptoms tell us that our gut health needs work. And it may sound dramatic, but unhealthy digestion can significantly impact other aspects of our well-being. So much so that when we face challenges with our skin or metabolism, one of the most critical steps to solve these issues is taking care of our digestive system.

Why is gut health so important?

Gut health refers to everything concerning the intestines, large and small bowels, and, most importantly, the condition of the microbiota or friendly bacteria. The gut, also called the digestive tract or the intestines, is the primary organ for nutrient absorption and waste elimination. It's also a huge hormone producer and controller. Researchers believe that the balance of the gut-brain axis, which is the gut's neural network, strongly affects a person's physiological and psychological health (Sun et al., 2020). Many consider our gut and its microbiome the foundations of our health. The gut is vital because it impacts digestion, immunity, the brain, hormones, and moods.

Women's and men's gut health also has significant differences. As women, we have different needs regarding our digestive system: we need more iron to support our monthly cycles, and we tend to experience symptoms like bloating more frequently. Moreover, we're generally at an increased risk of developing Irritable Bowel Syndrome (IBS). This risk may be caused by estrogen level fluctuations over time due to pregnancy and perimenopause or menopause transition years later in life.

Even among women, we each have unique needs because our bodies and how we want to look are different, so we need customized digestive health care. Most of the time, symptoms like acne, irritation, headache, and fatigue may go untreated and undiagnosed. These symptoms are common with poor digestive health.

So, if you're female and have been trying to get to that healthy place where your systems are finally in harmony, achieving balance in the digestive system is key. And to accomplish this, it's critical to truly understand this part of our body and customize our lifestyle, routine, diet, and supplements to target OUR concerns.

For example, let's take the term "IBS." You've likely heard it but may not fully understand what it entails. IBS is a common disorder that approximately 20% of Americans experience at some point. It's not a disease but a functional disorder affecting the digestive system. The symptoms can be chronic, including mild discomfort or severe abdominal pain, often accompanied by diarrhea or constipation. While it isn't a life-threatening disease, its symptoms are unpleasant.

There are many approaches to treating IBS, but these may not help everyone. Why? Because blindly following trends or taking supplements without understanding the root causes will rarely do any good. We need to properly understand how to treat IBS symptoms and other similar chronic conditions.

Having experienced gastrointestinal problems, I understand first-hand the struggles and frustrations of these issues. It isn't just about being unable to wear that fitted outfit because it feels uncomfortable when we're bloated or the embarrassment of passing gas. Aside from embarrassment and discomfort, more severe symptoms like diarrhea, constipation, and acid reflux will not only ruin a special event but may also impact health in other ways, such as damage to internal organs, malnourishment, pain, poor sleep, or skin problems.

My struggles have motivated me to learn more about these conditions to pinpoint the root cause and reach the ultimate goal: optimal digestive health free of all the symptoms that interfere with the full enjoyment of every moment of the day. Reaching that point, however, may not be that easy. While in the process of getting the book ready for publishing, I'm still trying different approaches in the hope that they will help to manage the symptoms.

So, why read this book in particular? If you're like me, suffering from chronic symptoms of unknown origin for a long time, this book contains information to help you understand the cause and the proper approach to manage its symptoms. A healthy gut can make all the difference for our body, mind, and spirit. Understanding this important system's anatomy and physiology can help us take proper steps toward recovery. In this book, aside from exploring the anatomy and physiology of our digestive tract, we'll look into the importance of our gut bacteria, the gut and brain connection, the basics of conventional disorders, including IBS, and how implementing dietary and lifestyle changes can help improve our symptoms.

1

THE GUT - ANATOMY, FUNCTIONS, AND SIGNIFICANCE

I t's fundamental that to begin understanding how our gut works, we need to know its anatomy—what parts make up this complex system and its physiology—and how those parts function together.

PARTS AND FUNCTIONS

The gastrointestinal tract begins in our mouth and ends in the anus. In between, there are essential organs. These include the esophagus, stomach, accessory organs such as the liver and pancreas, small intestine, appendix, and large intestine; parts of the large intestine are the cecum, colon, rectum, and anal canal.

Each part has a unique function, mostly related to digestion, but these organs also work together to manage other body needs. The digestive tract is a complex system, and no organ has one single function; instead, they have many effects that work like dominos that can set off or stop other reactions.

Let's go over some of the main digestive parts and their functions:

Mouth: The mouth grinds the food into a fine paste and mixes it with saliva. Saliva has amylase, an enzyme that starts the digestion of carbohydrates. We often hear that we must eat slowly because eating quickly and not letting the food mix with saliva may impair digestion.

Esophagus: The esophagus is a muscular tube that allows food to pass into the stomach to continue digestion and absorb nutrients. Not chewing food properly, trying to swallow a large amount, or eating sharp foods can easily tear the esophagus.

Stomach: The stomach is a muscular bag that stores food. It's here that food mixes with digestive juices. The stomach wall secretes hydrochloric acid (HCl), which helps digest proteins and converts pepsinogen to pepsin, an enzyme that breaks down protein. The stomach is our first defense against food-borne microbes such as salmonella or E. coli. The acidic environment kills most harmful microorganisms before they reach the intestines, where these microbes could cause severe damage to our health.

The stomach gradually empties food into the small intestine. This process could take up to four hours, depending on the type and amount of food we consume.

Small intestine: Most nutrients are absorbed here in the small intestine. There are fingerlike projections called villi that line its walls, and villi increase the surface area to improve nutrient absorption from food particles flowing through the intestine. It's also here where the absorption of vitamins occurs. However. this absorption may depend on other factors. For example, to absorb vitamin B12, a particular protein called the intrinsic factor produced in the stomach is needed, so if this process is impaired, it may result in B12 deficiency. Iron absorption requires vitamin C; therefore, a lack of vitamin C reduces the chances of absorbing this mineral, which is essential for the movement of oxygen throughout the body.

Substances produced in the liver and pancreas will also aid digestion in the small intestine. Bile production occurs in the liver and is released during the consumption of a fatty meal. Bile contains lecithin, an emulsifier that breaks down fat particles for more effective absorption. Bile will be stored in the gallbladder if there's no fat content to digest. Pancreatic juices are enzymes needed to digest fats and proteins and absorb fat-soluble vitamins like A, D, E, and K; these juices empty into the small intestine.

Large intestine: The main part of the large intestine is the colon, where water is absorbed back into our body after passing through the small intestine. Most water-soluble vitamins like vitamin C are absorbed here by cells lining the inner surface. It is also here where bacteria break down remaining indigestible matter like fiber, and as a result, it produces acids and gases.

Appendix: The appendix used to be considered a non-essential part of the gastrointestinal (GI) canal. However, our digestive system actually finds the appendix very useful. Its primary function is to act as a reservoir for beneficial bacteria to protect it from being flushed out when diarrhea or other intestinal problems occur.

THE SIGNIFICANCE OF GUT HEALTH

As explored in the previous section, the small intestine has a vast surface area for absorbing nutrients, and it serves as a barrier to harmful substances and microorganisms that may enter the body through food or water. In addition, our gut helps maintain homeostasis by producing hormones involved in appetite regulation, metabolism, and signals of satiety (the feeling of fullness after a meal).

The bacteria in our digestive tract help digest food molecules for better absorption through the intestines. These microbes also produce vitamin K, B12, and biotin for healthy growth and development. The gut flora also regulates the immune system by producing substances to help fight infections caused by pathogens or harmful microorganisms. This way, they help maintain intestinal integrity.

The gut is often called the second brain, as how we feel relates to what's happening in our digestive tract. Its own nervous system communicates with other body parts—including the brain—through hormones and nerve signals called neurotransmitters. This close relation is a direct contact called the "gut-brain axis." For example, suppose we're stressed out or anxious. A stressful mode may cause an increase in acid reflux or diarrhea because stress affects how the body processes food. Or sometimes, we might feel gloomy and depressed because of an imbalance in gut flora. The relationship is more direct than we would expect. Researchers have found that an imbalance in the digestive microbiome can cause cognitive impairment (Sun et al., 2020).

In summary, the gut also controls how much we eat, the absorption rate of all nutrients, and, to some degree, our happiness. These functions may seem a lot for a system concerned with eating, but that is why having a healthy gastrointestinal tract is so important.

BOWEL MOVEMENTS: AN INDICATOR OF DIGESTIVE HEALTH

So, how do we know if our gut is healthy? If we focus on our daily bowel movements, we can learn a lot about how optimal our digestive health is. Here are some signs from our bowel indicating ideal conditions in our GI tract:

Frequency: Generally, the ideal frequency of bowel movements is one daily, but most people have two to three daily passages. If you go more than three times a day or less than once a day, there may be a digestive problem.

Ease of passing: There shouldn't be straining during bowel movements. Needing to use force may indicate constipation or hemorrhoids.

Stool consistency: Stools should look like soft, long cylinders or logs, not loose or watery, but neither should they be hard or lumpy. Soft, regular-shaped stool indicates that our body absorbs enough water from food and that the intestines are properly moving waste through the digestive tract. The stools should also be brownish or yellowish in color. If they're black, blood may be passing, which is a problem.

Absence of diarrhea or constipation: Diarrhea occurs when stool moves too quickly through the intestines and causes water loss from the body. On the other hand, constipation occurs when stool moves too slowly through the intestines, causing them to harden in the colon (large intestine).

RECOGNIZING SIGNS OF POOR DIGESTIVE HEALTH

Sometimes, recognizing signs of adverse digestive health can be challenging because the symptoms we're experiencing may not always be related to our digestion.

Concerning digestive and non-digestive symptoms may include:

Upset stomach: Bloating, gas, and flatulence indicate a problem in our stomach. Certain foods potentially trigger these symptoms when our bodies can't digest them properly.

Food intolerance: If we have gut sensitivities, we may also experience digestive issues when consuming certain foods. When this occurs, we may also notice inflammation in the joints or skin (like acne), fatigue, or skin breakouts for no reason.

Conditions such as leaky gut syndrome: Leaky gut is also known as increased intestinal permeability, which refers to bacteria and toxins moving through the space between cells in the intestinal lining. Usually, a healthy intestinal wall would allow only nutrients to pass through into the bloodstream. But a defective membrane lets other particles in. Therefore, keeping this barrier intact is essential to help prevent foreign substances from crossing into the bloodstream. Unwanted substances in the blood can cause an immune response and trigger inflammation.

Sleep issues: Sleep problems are common alongside IBS or other digestive issues. Research shows that people with IBS have more difficulty falling and staying asleep than those without it. They also woke up more often at the night (Elsenbruch, 2005).

Skin rashes and allergies: Skin rashes are a common symptom of IBS. Researchers show that IBS patients are more prone to urticaria or hives, and 32% of females with IBS suffer skin rashes (Unal et al., 2018).

Sugar cravings: Poorly digested food will interfere with the balance of the gut's satiety process. So, despite eating enough, we often crave more because the gut can't communicate appropriately between its many parts and the brain. For example, a diet high in sugars could affect the balance of microbiota; balance is indispensable for proper brain-gut communication.

Autoimmune problems: Inadequate digestive health can also lead to an overabundance of harmful microorganisms in the digestive tract, which may trigger rheumatoid arthritis or thyroid issues.

Unexplained fatigue or sluggishness: If we feel tired all the time—even after a good night's sleep—it could be a sign of something wrong with our digestion. Fatigue is a common symptom of leaky gut, Irritable Bowel Disease (IBD), and IBS.

Unexplained mood disorders (i.e., depression or anxiety): The gut produces 90% of the serotonin, a neurotransmitter that regulates moods, so it should be no surprise that people with poor gut health often experience depression ("University of California," 2019) and anxiety.

Unexplained weight gain or weight loss: If you're trying to lose weight without success, consider whether impaired digestion may be affecting your metabolism and hormones in ways that aren't visible from the outside.

UNDERSTANDING THE UNIQUE DYNAMICS OF A WOMAN'S GUT

So, there are a lot of symptoms and problems for which the root cause lies in our GI tract, but we may not be aware of it. These symptoms differ from person to person. For example, a woman's gut behaves differently than a man's, and anatomy is the first and most apparent difference. The colon, the part of the intestinal tract closest to the rectum, is longer in women than in men. This difference means more room for bacteria to grow and flourish as food takes longer to pass through.

In addition to having more space for bacterial growth, female hormones also affect digestive health. Progesterone increases a specific bacterium in the intestine during pregnancy, preventing depression and anxiety. Estrogen also plays a vital role (Edwards et al., 2019). These hormones also change throughout a woman's life: childbirth, menopause, pregnancy, and aging.

These differences also vary in individual women based on their lifestyle, genetics, nationality, race, etc. Knowing which factors in our lives affect our gut the most is essential so that a restorative approach can be more effective.

———

Overall, all of the organs in our digestive tract have important interrelated functions essential for adequate digestion and absorption of nutrients and for their role in the gut and microbiome connection to the brain. Understanding our individual needs and how optimal or poor digestive health can manifest in our bodies is vital for us to adopt proper care.

2

GUT MICROBIOTA, SLEEP, AND WOMEN'S HORMONES

W e've discussed how the gut is a complex and fascinating organ responsible for many daily functions and behaviors. Digestion is its main function, but it also regulates hunger and releases hormones that influence our mood and emotions. It houses more than 70% of our body's immune cells. For these reasons, it's critical to maintain a healthy GI tract to prevent inflammation associated with many chronic illnesses and diseases.

A balanced gut flora or microbiome is the primary factor for optimal digestive functions.

The microbiome's composition in our digestive tract may differ depending on our lifestyle, food habits, and living conditions. Although slight differences wouldn't cause major illness, they will be enough to make us feel sick and tired and cause mild symptoms that we wouldn't be able to pinpoint the source of. For optimum health, we should focus on this significant bacterial colony.

EXPLORING THE FASCINATING GUT MICROBIOME

Our body contains ten times more bacteria than human cells, and 90% of these microbes live in our intestines. These bacteria living inside us are called the gut microbiota or gut microbiome.

Researchers estimate that more than 100 trillion bacteria reside in our digestive tract, which outnumbers human cells by 10 to 1. This complex system of microorganisms is now known to play an essential role in health and disease. This community includes bacteria, fungi, viruses, parasites, and other microbes, and together they weigh about 1 kg with 300-500 or more species variations (Rinninella et al., 2019). Just the weight shows how massive the amount is.

The gut microbiome has an important role: it helps us digest food, but it also produces vitamins, metabolizes nutrients, and converts these nutrients into energy for our bodies. The microbiome also regulates our immune system and protects us from harmful pathogens like salmonella and E. coli by producing antimicrobial chemicals called bacteriocins or by preventing them from attaching to the mucus lining of the gut wall. They also affect our mood and behavior.

In relationship to our microbiota's role in immunity, there is a strong association between specific types of gut bacteria and conditions such as IBD and others (Qiu et al., 2022).

HOW THE GUT MICROBIOME TAKES SHAPE:

Our intestinal microbiome is established at birth and, after that, is affected by breastfeeding, genetics, age, gender, and other possible factors. The composition of the gut flora changes throughout our life—for example, as babies, we have relatively few species but acquire more over time.

These factors come into play and have an impact on our microbiota:

Gestational age and the delivery method: A vaginal birth exposes the baby to more bacteria. Hence, the baby acquires more species in its gut microbiome. Similarly, babies born at full term tend to have higher and more diverse microbiota.

Milk feeding methods: Whether the baby drinks breast milk or formula milk also affects the composition and diversity of the gut microbiome. Research indicates that Lactoferrin (LF) in a mother's milk influences neonatal microbiota creation and development, contributing to the baby's immunology. This immunology is more important in preterm babies (Mastromarino et al., 2014).

Age and use of antibiotics: Some bacteria become more prominent as others die because of certain antibiotics or as we age. Antibiotics could very quickly cause a microbiome imbalance. The condition of our microbiome can affect how we age. As we age, our intestinal flora becomes less diverse, and good bacteria are replaced by unfriendly microorganisms. In a study, researchers found that people with more varied microbiomes tended to live healthier and longer than those with less diversity in their microbiota ("Unique Gut Microbiome," 2021).

Diet: The other factor that enhances the microbiome in later life is diet. A high-fiber diet produces more varieties of bacteria species. On the contrary, diets rich in fats, sugar, and animal protein can disrupt the microbiome's balance and reduce its diversity.

MICROBIOTA VS MICROBIOME

The term microbiome is used interchangeably with microbiota. However, note some differences in their meaning.

A microbiome usually comprises many different microorganism species, their genes, and the environmental factors that influence them. So, when referring to the microbiome, scientists refer to the entire microorganisms and the "home" where these microorganisms live.

A microbiota, on the other hand, is a specific group of microbes found within an environment or on a host organism. Microbiota refers to all the microorganisms, including bacteria, viruses, fungi, and protozoa, living in or on an organism or its environment, such as soil. For example, our gut microbiota includes all microorganisms inside our intestines.

MICROBIOTA AND GUT HEALTH

As we know now, several factors determine the types of bacteria that live in our intestine, including how we were born, where we were born (village or city), our food as babies (breastmilk vs. formula), and how long we breastfed (1 year or less). When we're young, the types of bacteria change very quickly; however, as we grow older, our microbiota becomes more stable.

The microbiota has different species, many of which aren't permanent. The transient species consists of opportunistic microbes that enter the body through food, water, or other contact. These species are generally less abundant than their stable counterparts. Stable microbiota inhabits our intestines, skin, and respiratory tract. They maintain homeostasis within these tissues by regulating immune responses to pathogens and preserving tissue integrity.

Studies show that Bacteroidetes and Firmicutes bacteria are the dominant species in our GI tract, along with other types like Actinobacteria, Proteobacteria, and Verrucomicrobia. These microorganisms' presence conserves optimal health (Lozupone et al., 2012). According to Dr. Lozupone and his team, balancing the gut microbiota is like keeping a well-maintained lawn. The harmful bacteria, or the "weeds," must be plucked out or kept under control, and the good bacteria and microorganisms, or the "grass," must be fed regularly. Otherwise, the grass will die, and the weeds will grow in its place, ruining the lawn.

Here's how a well-balanced and diverse gut microbiota benefits our health:

Digestion and immune support: These microbes help digest food, extract nutrients, and metabolize those nutrients. In addition, they affect the host-regulated adaptive immune system that has a role in reacting only to harmful substances; when this process fails, our system can attack itself, which can result in autoimmune diseases (Zhang et al., 2014).

Nutrient metabolism and protection: The gut microbiota metabolizes carbohydrates, especially fiber, into metabolites our body can absorb. It also helps us absorb iron, calcium, and other minerals. It produces natural antibiotics called bacteriocins that help us fight off pathogens like salmonella or E. Coli, which may cause food poisoning.

Inflammatory and anti-tumor activity: Our microbiota can regulate inflammation by producing short-chain fatty acids (SCFAs) during the fermentation of complex carbohydrates in the colon. These SCFAs also have potential anti-tumor properties.

Impact on cancer therapy: Research shows patients going through immunochemotherapy, bone marrow recipients, and those with autoimmune diseases could experience significant changes in recovery response when their gut microbiota is balanced (Alexander et al., 2017). A diverse microbiome can improve the response to anticancer procedures. Unfortunately, these methods often result in disruption to the microbiota.

Fiber breakdown and obesity prevention: The microbiota helps process fiber, one of the primary energy sources for the cells lining the small intestine. Dietary fiber can help us feel satiated faster, and this can help reduce the risk of obesity.

DISRUPTION OF GUT MICROBIOTA

Maintaining a proper pH (acid/alkaline balance) in the intestines is critical for a balanced microbiota and protecting against diseases.

In addition to the importance of pH, several factors can alter the balance of the microbiome. The first is diet. The microbiota of someone who eats a diet high in sugar and processed foods will differ from that of someone who eats a diet high in fresh fruits and vegetables. Not only do different foods contain or produce different bacteria, as in the case of fermented food, but food can also nourish the bacteria. A diet high in sugar will disrupt the microbiota, where harmful bacteria may outnumber friendly types. For example, yeast, a fungus, can become unbalanced and grow out of control as it thrives in a sugary environment.

Stress and smoking can affect microbiota composition. Stress can cause variations in our gut flora due to changes in blood flow to the digestive tract, while smoking may decrease diversity.

Some diseases are also known to change our microbiota composition because they damage or destroy certain types of bacteria. For example, Crohn's disease causes changes due to the autoimmune reactions it induces.

Antibiotics can also have an impact. Antibiotics fight off infections by removing the microorganisms that cause them. But these drugs are a double-edged sword. They can be lifesaving and remedy infections but also kill off good bacteria.

Moreover, antibiotics aren't just for us humans—they're also used on farms and in animal feedlots, which means they're present in our food supply at almost every stage of its production. So, we're constantly taking them, harming our microflora balance.

SLEEP AND GUT MICROBIOTA

According to recent research, gut bacteria can influence our sleep quality. Similarly, sleep quality can affect bacteria diversity in the intestines (Neroni et al., 2021).

Gut microbes produce neurotransmitters serotonin, dopamine, melatonin, and GABA (gamma-aminobutyric acid), among others. These substances ensure a good night's sleep and that we feel rested when we wake up. If our digestive microbes aren't healthy, we may not be able to get enough restorative sleep—and when that happens, our immunity drops, and we become more susceptible to illness and disease. We would also be more likely to feel moody or anxious while awake.

Scientists found that people with IBS or GERD are prone to more disrupted sleep than people without those conditions.

Considering what researchers have found about our gut microbiome affecting sleep, it makes sense that manipulating the intestinal flora is now considered a therapeutic approach for sleep disorders. In one study on mice, researchers discovered that probiotics helped them improve sleep quality and reduced anxiety and stress levels while they slept (Thompson et al., 2017).

Recent studies have also shown that certain bacteria can lead to better sleep. Scientists noted that people with higher Bacteroides fragilis and bifidobacterium levels experienced more restful sleep (Wang et al., 2022). These bacteria most likely regulate sleep by modulating how the brain controls chemical processes.

However, whether these findings also apply to humans is still unclear. Nonetheless, this research gives insight into how our gut bacteria affect the brain and body!

THE GUT MICROBIOME'S ROLE IN HORMONAL BALANCE

One study pointed out the ovary and adrenal glands aren't the only organs that produce estrogen. But one of the central regulators of estrogen is our gut microbiome (Baker et al., 2017). Estrobolome is the term for all the genes in the gut microbiome that influence estrogen production. Estrobolome genes are involved in everything from metabolism to inflammation and play a huge role in female reproductive health. It secretes β-glucuronidase, which acts as an enzyme that activates estrogen. Then, these active estrogen particles can be absorbed into the circulation and taken up by target cells throughout the body. β-glucuronidase also breaks down complex carbohydrates and aids in absorbing flavonoids (substances with antioxidant properties) and bilirubin (a byproduct of the destruction of old red blood cells). When the microbiota is healthy, it helps to remove the extra estrogen via stool and urine, preventing cancer and other hormonal imbalances.

THE CONNECTION BETWEEN GUT HEALTH, HORMONAL IMBALANCE, AND PCOS

Estrogen-related diseases like polycystic ovarian syndrome (PCOS), endometriosis, and breast cancer are often the result of poor digestive health.

Researchers believe impaired digestion's effects create an environment where an imbalance in estrogen can be produced (Baker et al., 2017). This imbalance can lead to irregular menstrual cycles and infertility in women with PCOS. In women with endometriosis, the excess estrogen can cause pain during menstruation and extreme bleeding during periods.

PCOS, especially, can be very severe on our health. This hormonal condition affects many of us, and the cause may be an imbalance of sex hormones: an excess of androgen, a male sex hormone, leading to small ovary cysts. The symptoms of PCOS include irregular menstrual periods, acne, hirsutism (excessive face and body hair), weight gain, and ovarian cysts.

Combined with gut dysbiosis, PCOS is a multifaceted disease affecting many bodily areas, not just the ovaries. Insulin resistance is common in people with PCOS (Diamanti-Kandarakis et al., 2009). This disorder causes blood sugar levels to rise above standard levels. In the long term, elevated levels of blood sugar can lead to nerve damage, blindness, and kidney failure. They also increase the risk of breast and uterine cancer.

To summarize, our gastrointestinal tract's community of microorganisms, or the microbiome, impacts our health. Established at birth, this community protects us from harmful microbes and aids our immune system. A balanced microbiome is essential for good digestion, emotional health, sleep, and hormonal balance.

3

UNDERSTANDING THE GUT-BRAIN CONNECTION

The connection between our gut and brain occurs in many ways, and it's crucial to understand how this connection works. Our complex nervous system includes parts of the brain, spinal cord, and several large nerves. These components connect the brain and the gut, and this system controls everything from our heartbeat to our digestion.

This strong gut and brain connection oversees much of our health and immensely affects our mood and overall wellness. The two work together to keep each other healthy by sending signals back and forth through the nervous system. When one or both systems don't appropriately receive these signals, there could be severe consequences for our mental or physical health—or both!

Experiencing stress or trauma can cause physical changes in the brain, leading to chronic illnesses like depression and heart disease.

WHAT'S INVOLVED IN THE GUT-BRAIN CONNECTION?

The gut is considered a second brain for several reasons. For example, our intestines contain more neurons than our spinal cord and have an independent nervous system.

The gut-brain axis is a structure of complex connections between the GI tract and the central nervous system, regulating numerous processes in our body. The microbiota influences the immune system, hormones, and central nervous system. Changes that occur during these interactions are then communicated to the brain. It's like a two-way street: brain activity affects the microbiome, but the microbiome changes also affect brain function. There are several ways these mechanisms are achieved. The central nervous system or brain sends signals to the intestines via fibers in the vagus nerve (a cranial nerve that controls other organs and body functions), causing changes in gut motility and the secretion of hormones such as serotonin.

The gastrointestinal tract uses neurotransmitters, chemical substances that carry messages between nerve cells. These substances help regulate mood, sleep, and appetite. Dopamine, serotonin, acetylcholine, and GABA neurotransmitters are essential in mood regulation and affect anxiety levels. Our microbiota can influence these neurotransmitters by increasing or decreasing their production in our body or altering how they function once they reach the brain. GABA acts on the brainstem to suppress vagal nerve activity (Carabotti et al., 2015). The production of serotonin also affects the brain and will provide calming effects at the appropriate levels.

Additionally, microorganisms in the gastrointestinal tract produce metabolites. These substances alter host gene expression and signaling pathways involved in inflammation and metabolism.

Motility is how quickly food moves along our intestine, and a significant way that the brain affects the gut is via intestinal motility through the vagus nerve. The vagus nerve runs from the brainstem, reaching the abdomen. Among other functions, it controls the muscles moving food through the digestive tract. For example, swallowing food stimulates nerves in our mouth that send signals to the brain, telling the stomach muscles to contract (squeeze). Then, those muscles squeeze together to push food into the small intestine. Another way the brain can affect how quickly food travels through the intestines is by controlling secretion from cells lining the intestinal wall (Carabotti et al., 2015).

When stressed, the brain, gut motility, and secretions are affected. That's why sometimes, we may feel nauseous or experience other digestive symptoms if we're facing negative situations.

There's a relationship between imbalances in the microbiome and conditions like IBD, IBS, and Parkinson's disease.

According to studies, gastrointestinal inflammation has a connection to the mental decline in Alzheimer's disease (AD), Parkinson's disease (PD), and Huntington's disease (Günther et al., 2021). AD is thought to be associated with intestinal dysbiosis (a microbial imbalance in the gut). In short, the inflammation in the intestines due to dysbiosis and the resulting inflammatory and immune reaction may be the underlying cause of many neurodegenerative diseases. Particles that cross the intestinal membrane then cross the blood-brain barrier and can cause different inflammatory responses in the brain, leading to Alzheimer's and similar disorders.

THE NEUROTRANSMITTERS

The enteric nervous system's (ENS) responsibility is to regulate the work of the gastrointestinal tract. In addition to food digestion, absorption, and secretion, the ENS controls immune functions, body temperature, and blood pressure.

The ENS has neurotransmitters regulating intestinal contractions, secretions, and motility. Some neurotransmitters, like serotonin, are mostly produced in the intestines. Also, in the intestines, gut neurons release dopamine, GABA, and noradrenaline into the bloodstream. These substances can then act in the brain via projections of the vagus nerves, which connect the gastrointestinal tract to various parts of the brain, including areas involved in mood control.

Additionally, researchers also found that microbiome bacteria can consume neurotransmitters as well as produce them. So, our microbiota can increase and decrease the neurotransmitter level. Neurotransmitters are how the sympathetic (fight or flight response) and parasympathetic (rest and digest) nervous systems control several bodily functions. So, this control has a significant effect on the overall body.

The three significant effects of the neurotransmitters released by the gut microbiome are:

Activation of the HPA axis: The hypothalamic-pituitary-adrenal (HPA) axis is a significant neuroendocrine stress response process and coordinates the body's physiological responses to stressors. When these processes are continually activated, as occurs if we're constantly under a lot of stress, it can lead to various physiological disturbances, including fatigue, depression, anxiety, and sleep troubles.

Host neurotransmitter catabolism: Evidence suggests that our microbiota affects serotonin metabolism in several ways, including the direct effects on the expression of genes responsible for synthesizing and breaking down molecules where microbial enzymes or other processes are involved.

Innervation via the vagus nerve: The vagus nerve is part of a much more significant effect the intestinal tract exerts.

THE VAGUS NERVE

The vagus nerve, one of our body's most elongated cranial nerves, starts in the brain, travels down to the chest, abdomen, and pelvis, and branches out to different organs. It's also the only cranial nerve that travels to low parts of the body and controls most organs and bodily functions.

The most critical role of this nerve is to balance the parasympathetic nervous system, which controls functions when our body is at rest. Some of the effects of an activated parasympathetic nervous system are a slowdown of the heart, a speed-up of digestion, a slowdown of breathing, a drop in blood pressure, smaller pupils, and the relaxing of the eyes.

The vagus nerve is considered the sixth sense in interoceptive awareness (capacity to identify, access, understand, and respond accordingly to the pattern of internal signals). It means it communicates information about the body's state to the brain. This nerve may also be responsible for facilitating our sense of intuition. This belief is a hypothesis from many scientists that the sixth sense might be mediated by the right vagus nerve, which connects with the pituitary gland: the master gland that controls almost all hormone secretions.

Because of the connection to our gut microbiome, the vagus nerve can sense the metabolites produced by the bacteria there. Then, it transfers this information to the central nervous system for integration into the central autonomic network. And finally, it generates an adapted or inappropriate response. Inappropriate responses are rare. But, if present, this can result in digestive and neurodegenerative disorders.

The vagus nerve has control over the gut microbiome environment. It prevents inflammation through the cholinergic anti-inflammatory pathway, which is another part of the ANS. But, stress can inhibit this pathway and harm the gastrointestinal tract and our microbiota, resulting in gastrointestinal disorders. In addition, this nerve controls hunger/satiety, stress responses, and inflammation to certain degrees.

Studies show elevated inflammatory markers, also called cytokines, are associated with a higher chance of suffering from disorders like schizophrenia, bipolar disorder, major depression, and obsessive-compulsive disorder (Kirkpatrick et al., 2013).

STRESS

Stress is a natural element of life, and we all react differently. Some of us shrug it off, while others may get wound up.

The latter reaction is common among people with disorders affecting the gastrointestinal tract. Stress can profoundly affect digestion, causing abdominal pain, diarrhea, constipation, nausea, vomiting, and other digestive symptoms. And these problems can occur even when the gut isn't technically affected by the disease. Everything around us becomes more significant when stressed— our survival depends on it. And this is good when there's an immediate threat, but if stress becomes chronic, the body can start to experience wide-ranging effects that make us unhealthy.

Stress stimulates the sympathetic (the fight or flight response) nervous system, which inhibits the vagus nerve. Suppressing the vagal nerve can cause microbiota alterations, triggering GI issues.

The second way stress affects digestion is by causing changes to the bacteria in our intestines. Some bacteria are eaten by others when the vagus and anti-inflammatory functions aren't working, which throws the balance off.

KEEPING A HEALTHY MICROBIOME

To keep our gut microbiome in good shape, we must deal with stress without depending on unhealthy habits like smoking, eating junk food, or taking painkillers. Establishing practices to deal with stressful situations is vital for our overall health.

One effective way to manage stress levels is to increase physical activity. Exercise increases blood flow and circulation, which is necessary for the body to effectively remove waste products and other harmful substances from the bloodstream. A quick walk or doing stretches will work wonders to reduce stress.

Alongside exercise, an adequate diet that includes healthy proteins, fats, and plenty of fruits and vegetables is necessary. These foods are high in nutrients and antioxidants, which help protect cells from impairment caused by free radicals (harmful substances in our body), which would otherwise cause inflammation and contribute to leaky-gut syndrome, for example. A diet high in fiber will also help our microbiome.

Another easy way to reduce stress response is with meditation. Meditation allows us to step back from stressful situations and gain perspective.

We can learn to identify stressful situations before they occur and become proactive in reducing or preventing them altogether.

Probiotic supplements can help remodel our gut microbiome, making it more resilient against the harmful effects of stress.

In later chapters, we will explore more in-depth stress-reducing techniques, food approaches, and supplementation.

As we've seen, there's a strong relationship between the gut and the brain; interactions called the gut-brain axis. These interactions, which stress can impact, help regulate most bodily functions, including metabolism and inflammation. We need to take steps to keep a healthy microbiome.

4

THE UNIQUENESS OF GUT HEALTH-ASSOCIATED DISORDERS

A s the saying goes, *"All disease begins in the gut"* (Hippocrates).

Imbalances in our digestive microbiota are often associated with disorders involving inflammation, permeability, poor motility, or food sensitivities. Each condition is unique. For example, some of us might have a leaky gut, and others might have IBS. So, knowing how these diseases manifest in our bodies is essential for taking the proper steps to address the symptoms and find relief.

SIBO

Small Intestine Bacterial Overgrowth (SIBO) happens when bacteria levels are abnormal in the small intestine. Under normal conditions, bacteria in this part of our digestive tract should be minimal compared to that in the large intestine. With SIBO, toxins can be produced, interfering with digestion and nutrient absorption and resulting in diarrhea, constipation, or other digestive symptoms (Dukowicz et al., 2007).

Two types of SIBO have been identified: hydrogen and methane.

The hydrogen type occurs when there are too many hydrogen-producing bacteria. The belief is that this type of bacteria is commonly associated with diarrhea symptoms. The hydrogen SIBO diagnosis is by identifying elevated hydrogen levels in a breath test.

Methane SIBO occurs when there are too many methane-producing bacteria. This occurrence is usually associated with constipation. High methane levels on the breath test indicate a positive diagnosis for this type of SIBO.

In addition to diagnosing SIBO through a breath test, another method used is the extraction of intestinal fluid through an endoscopy to determine the growth of bacteria in the small intestine.

Causes:

Several factors can lead to SIBO:

An impaired migrating motor complex (MMC): The MMC are muscle contractions or a cleaning mechanism responsible for the movement of remaining matter in the stomach and intestines. This motility process takes place in between eating or in a fasting state. If this mechanism is slow or damaged, it creates an environment where food fermentation occurs, and bacteria can thrive, leading to symptoms that include gas, bloating, constipation, or diarrhea. It's worth noting that this mechanism isn't the same as peristalsis, which moves food through the digestive tract and is triggered when we eat. The MMC occurs about one hour and a half after consuming food; it occurs in several phases when we aren't eating and may last about two hours.

Inhibited enzymes, bile, and gastric acid: Gastric acid prevents bacteria from reaching the small intestine; enzymes break food down to improve absorption, and bile breaks down fats. An imbalance of these components can compromise digestion and provide bacteria with an ideal environment to multiply more quickly.

Complications of abdominal surgery: Surgical procedures such as gastric bypass or those to treat stomach ulcers can impair motility or create spaces where bacteria accumulate.

Structural problems in the small intestine: For example, scarred tissue or pouches or diverticula that bulge through the walls of the intestine (typical in diverticulosis cases) can result in the slow movement of food, which may lead to fermentation and bacterial overgrowth.

Gastrointestinal conditions such as IBS and diabetes: Studies indicate a connection between SIBO and insulin levels. In such studies, SIBO patients were found to have higher glucose levels. Similarly, a strong link exists between SIBO and IBS, such that about 80% of people who suffer from IBS also have SIBO (Yan et al.,2020). These two conditions are related and share similar symptoms. Some may think SIBO is the cause of IBS, and others, on the contrary, that IBS causes SIBO.

Overuse of antibiotics and antiacid-blocking medications: Antibiotics destroy beneficial and harmful bacteria. This damage can create an imbalance or an overgrowth of harmful microorganisms.

Symptoms:

The presence of SIBO can be identified via symptoms such as:

- Bloating, constipation, diarrhea
- Feeling of fullness after eating
- Abdominal pain and loss of appetite
- Nausea
- Weight loss and malnutrition

Complications:

Treating SIBO is vital to avoid serious health complications:

- Nutritional deficiencies caused by the impairment in the absorption of nutrients
- Osteoporosis and kidney stones due to the poor absorption of calcium
- Occasionally restless leg syndrome, interstitial cystitis, rosacea, and psoriasis
- IBS patients can have a high prevalence of SIBO. In about two-thirds of cases, IBS is related to or caused by

SIBO (more in the IBS-D type-diarrhea type). The symptoms for both conditions can be similar; however, there are clinical tests to determine the presence of bacterial overgrowth, while IBS is a disorder diagnosed based only on the assessment of symptoms.

Therapeutic Approach:

SIBO recovery is a multi-step approach. Identifying and addressing the underlying cause is essential, as well as supporting and maintaining long-term digestive health.

From a diet standpoint, one approach to control the symptoms of SIBO is "starving" the bacteria involved in the overgrowth. This task is accomplished by reducing or eliminating fermentable food sources, as these foods tend to cause gas, bloating, diarrhea, or constipation. Fermentable foods, which can also be known as FODMAPs (Fermentable Oligosaccharides, Disaccharides, Monosaccharides, and Polyols), include grains, fruits, certain vegetables, dairy, and legumes.

Refer in the next chapter to list of high and low FODMAP foods.

Another tip is to consume more cooked foods and limit snacking. Cooked foods tend to be easier for our body to digest, and this will improve the absorption of nutrients. Avoiding snacking or continuous eating will let digestion rest between meals, allowing our motor mechanism or MMC to activate and remove residual food or bacteria from our stomach and intestines, thus preventing fermentation.

The types of foods and how often we consume them will play an essential role in treating the symptoms of SIBO; however, addressing the root cause is critical. Both types of SIBO, methane or hydrogen, can be remediated with natural antibiotics and antimicrobials.

For hydrogen-type SIBO, consider taking herbal remedies like berberine, neem oil, oregano oil, and guar gum.

The therapeutical method for methane-SIBO includes remedies like allicin (garlic) formulas, oregano oil, and neem leaf extract.

Poor motility can be addressed with supplements or prokinetics formulas to improve these processes. 5HTP (5-hydroxytryptophan, made from tryptophan amino acid, which the body can convert to serotonin), ginger, peppermint oil, and Triphala are considered beneficial.

Combining and rotating between these protocols is recommended to avoid bacterial resistance. The approach with these natural antibiotics should last 30 to 60 days, depending on the bacteria levels.

Taking digestive enzymes, hydrochloric acid, and fish oil supplements is essential for the continued support of our digestive health. Vitamins (B12, A, D, and K), minerals (magnesium, zinc, iron, calcium, and copper), prebiotics, and probiotics are also necessary.

CANDIDA

Candida is a fungus or yeast typically found on the skin, mouth, throat, gut, and vagina. This fungus is part of our microbiota. But if there's an overgrowth, it can cause candidiasis or yeast infections. It can also cause dangerous blood infections if it crosses the intestinal epithelial barrier.

More than 20 types of candida have possibly been identified to cause candidiasis; the most common is Candida albicans. These infections can happen to anyone with a weakened immune system. Women are more prone to this condition, especially those with uncontrolled blood sugar or a poor immune system.

Candidiasis is usually harmless but can be severe when occurring in the intestine. Research may indicate that C. Albicans infection increases intestinal barrier permeability and promotes the movement of bacteria and bacterial products into the blood (Allert et al., 2018).

The presence of candida is diagnosed by taking a sample of the affected area, endoscopy, or blood or stool test.

Causes:

Several things can cause candida to grow out of control:

Imbalanced microbiota: The microorganisms in the gut and mouth can significantly impact how well our immune system functions. When they aren't in balance, it can lead to an overgrowth of yeast.

Antibiotics: Taking antibiotics for an extended period increases the risk of candida overgrowth, as antibiotics will also harm beneficial bacteria. Damage to the gut flora can leave open space for pathogens like Candida albicans to take hold and multiply quickly.

Compromised immune system: A compromised immune system is more vulnerable to developing candida overgrowth because the body can't fight off infections as well as it should.

Diabetes: A diabetes condition increases the risk of a person suffering from candida infections, likely due to increased blood sugar levels that feed the growth of these microorganisms, making it more challenging to treat candidiasis.

Symptoms:

When candida invades the body, it can manifest in several ways. Some of the most common symptoms include:

- Oral thrush, a condition where fungus grows on the tongue or mouth
- Fatigue
- Urinary and genital infections
- Digestive disorders, including bloating, constipation, cramps, diarrhea, gasses, nausea
- Joint pain
- Sinus infections
- Skin and nail fungal infections

Complications:

Candida complications are dangerous and can be life-threatening if not treated quickly. Invasive candidiasis, for example, is a condition that occurs when candida enters the bloodstream and invades other body parts.

These are possible complications:

- Fever that lasts longer than three days
- Chills accompanied by a cough or belly pain
- Low blood pressure
- Muscle aches
- Skin rash
- Weakness or fatigue
- Invasive candidiasis infection can also cause more specific symptoms, such as:

  o Blurriness in the eyes caused by an eye infection
  o Headaches caused by an infection in the brain

Therapeutical Approach:

Reducing carbohydrates in our diet can help to stop the yeast from growing. These types of food include sugar, gluten-containing foods like bread and pasta, alcohol, dairy products (especially cheese), mushrooms, fermented foods, and vinegar-based condiments like mustard and salad dressings.

These other dietary tips are recommended: avoid processed foods with added sugar, salt, and preservatives; reduce fruit consumption and focus on consuming leafy greens, cruciferous and non-starchy vegetables, cooked foods, lean proteins, and healthy fats.

To clear candidiasis naturally, include natural antibiotics and antimicrobials like berberine, colloidal silver, caprylic acid, mastic gum, and oregano oil.

Boric acid suppositories can be efficient in treating yeast infections.

Other natural remedies for preventing and maintaining a healthy digestive balance are coconut oil, bone broth, and lemon water. Probiotics also help restore beneficial bacteria in our intestines.

Liver support supplements such as milk thistle help reduce inflammation and bolster the liver's ability to detoxify byproducts from the body's metabolic processes.

Multivitamins/minerals and omega-3 fatty acids are also essential for overall health and for managing candida outbreaks.

LEAKY GUT

Leaky gut syndrome, or intestinal permeability, is a condition where undigested food or other harmful particles can pass through the defective lining in our intestine into the tissue below and the bloodstream. Damage to the intestinal membrane occurs when gaps or holes in the lining become wider, thus making the membrane more porous. Bacteria can cause damage and weaken this protective layer. This permeability allows large molecules to pass through. Under a normal absorption process, only nutrients from the food broken down by digestive enzymes should be allowed to cross the intestinal barrier into the bloodstream (Allan et al., 2022).

When undigested food particles or other substances enter the bloodstream, they may trigger an immune response and inflammation. In addition to causing inflammation in the gastrointestinal tract and contributing to digestive disorders, some believe a leaky gut may have a connection to depression and anxiety.

Leaky gut isn't currently recognized as a medical condition despite growing evidence suggesting potentially far-reaching effects on health.

Causes:

The cause of leaky gut is often chronic inflammation, celiac disease, and bacterial imbalances. Other causes include:

- Chemotherapy procedures
- Stress or trauma to the digestive system
- Intestinal injury from surgery or other causes
- Food allergies
- Chronic infections like candida or parasites

Symptoms:

Symptoms are often similar to other digestive conditions. These include:

- Diarrhea, constipation, and bloating
- Nutritional deficiencies
- Fatigue
- Headaches
- Skin problems and joint pain
- Inflammation
- Hormonal imbalances

Complications:

A leaky gut can result in many complications, the most common being fibromyalgia, chronic fatigue syndrome, asthma, and autoimmune diseases like diabetes and arthritis. It's important to note that a leaky gut isn't the cause of these conditions—it's a symptom, or the same condition that causes these is also causing a leaky gut.

Therapeutical Approach:

One step in fixing leaky gut is to identify food allergens. This identification can be done through a blood test or by carefully tracking symptoms throughout the day and eliminating foods that cause the problems. Some common allergenic foods include wheat in many bread types, dairy and soy products, nuts and seeds, eggs, corn, and legumes.

Once the trigger foods are identified, they should be eliminated or minimized, and we can then focus instead on consuming safer options. These include high-fiber foods—plenty of fruits and vegetables, organic grass-fed meats, healthy fats, and fermented foods.

We should avoid refined foods with additives that can potentially be allergens; a diet high in processed foods also negatively affects the diversity of our gut microbiome.

Dietary approaches considered helpful are a low FODMAP, a paleo diet, or intermittent fasting. These diets can help repair leaky gut by reducing inflammation in the GI tract while repairing damage caused by food allergens.

In addition to following anti-inflammatory diets, certain supplements can be beneficial. Some examples are probiotics, amino acids such as L-glutamine, minerals like zinc, and healthy oils like omega-3. These supplements help repair damage and help keep the immune system strong. Multivitamins and bone broth are rich in nutrients and help replenish deficient nutrients due to poor absorption. Digestive enzymes will aid in properly breaking down proteins, fats, and carbohydrates to improve nutrient absorption. Herbal remedies like licorice, turmeric, marshmallow root, Pau D'arco, oregano oil, and slippery elm can soothe and support the intestinal lining.

CELIAC DISEASE

It is an autoimmune disease triggered by consuming foods containing gluten. This immune response damages the small intestine lining, leading to an inability to absorb nutrients.

Celiac disease can be diagnosed with a blood test or a biopsy.

Causes:

Although gluten is the main trigger of celiac disease, there may be other factors:

Gluten: Gluten, a protein in wheat, barley, and rye, holds food particles together and gives food a stretchable consistency, like a piece of dough. In our intestines, cell receptors identify this protein as harmful, and an inflammatory response causes damage to the intestinal barrier. This abnormal immune response to gluten is the leading cause of celiac disease.

Genes: Some people inherit genes that make them more susceptible to developing this condition. Having one or more first-degree relatives (parents or siblings) diagnosed with celiac disease puts us at a higher risk of getting it. But even if no one in the family has it, developing the condition is possible if other factors are involved—like certain infections or lifestyle choices.

Gut dysbiosis: Gut dysbiosis, or the imbalance of bacteria in our intestine, causes inflammation, which leads to damage to the intestinal lining and, ultimately, an inability to absorb nutrients properly and possibly developing a susceptibility to gluten.

Infections: Certain gastrointestinal infections can trigger an autoimmune response that may result in celiac disease.

Type 1 diabetes: There is a link between this condition and celiac disease, possibly because both are autoimmune disorders. Type 1 diabetes, therefore, increases the risk of suffering celiac disease.

Symptoms:

The symptoms of celiac disease can differ from person to person. While some people may not experience any symptoms, others may experience malnutrition and osteoporosis due to the impaired absorption from an inflamed intestine.

Other symptoms are similar to other digestive conditions:

- Bloating, constipation, diarrhea, gas
- Lactose intolerance
- Abdominal pain
- Smelly and greasy stool
- Nausea or vomiting

Complications:

Celiac disease can cause several complications due to poor absorption.

Anemia: This is a common complication when iron or vitamin B12 is low. This deficiency can lead to pale skin, tiredness, weakness, shortness of breath, and heart palpitations. Treating cases of anemia with iron supplements and vitamin B12 is essential.

Osteoporosis: Osteoporosis is a bone-thinning disorder that affects bone density and strength caused by the low calcium levels in the blood. Osteoporosis is rare in people younger than 40 but is more common in people older than 60. In general, women tend to have low levels of vitamin D; therefore, supplementing with a daily dose is essential for prevention.

Nervous system issues: These could include symptoms such as numbness in the hands and feet, poor balance, difficulty walking straight, confusion, memory loss, and mood changes like depression and anxiety.

Joint pain: Joint pain is common in people with celiac disease because of inflammation affecting the joints' synovial membrane. It causes swelling around the joints, leading to knee or ankle stiffness, making it hard to walk correctly or when standing up straight.

Skin problems: Skin problems like breakouts, urticaria, and psoriasis can occur.

Heart, liver, and gallbladder problems: The lack of nutrients because of the poor absorption in the intestines can cause damage to these organs. Not to mention, a damaged intestinal barrier allows toxins to pass through, which overloads the liver and may result in liver impairment over time. The inflammation response triggered by gluten can impact the heart, the hardening of the arteries, and cause plaque formation. One possible situation that affects the gallbladder is that hormones in the intestine don't work correctly. Therefore, there's an impairment of signals to the gallbladder to release enzymes for the digestion of fats, resulting in the formation of gallstones.

Impact on pancreas and spleen: Excessive inflammation stresses the spleen, which filters blood contents. In addition, low levels of nutrients like folate could also damage this organ. Gluten particles in the pancreas may inappropriately stimulate insulin secretion.

Therapeutical Approach:

A strict gluten-free diet is necessary for treating celiac disease and preventing further damage to the intestinal barrier. Gluten proteins are in wheat, rye, barley, and other grains.

Along with a diet free of gluten, other recommendations include:

Avoid unexpected sources of gluten. Everyday household items like toothpaste and mouthwash may contain it because barley-based alcohol or other food additives derived from wheat are components of these products. Over-the-counter medications/supplements may also contain gluten, so checking any medications before taking them is important ("Celiac Disease," 2022).

Take multivitamins/minerals. Because nutritional deficiencies are common, supplementing is needed to get all the nutrients not absorbed from food sources alone. The most frequent deficiencies are vitamin B12, folic acid, iron, zinc, and vitamin D.

Include digestive enzymes or probiotics if there are issues digesting certain foods like dairy. Enzymes help break down food to improve absorption in the intestine and help strengthen digestive health overall. Probiotics will assist in restoring the microbiota.

Fish oil could be beneficial if included in our daily routine. Essential fatty acid levels are usually low in patients with celiac disease due to low absorption and high levels of inflammation.

IBD

Inflammatory Bowel Disease (IBD) is a lifelong condition characterized by inflammation in the gastrointestinal tract. It can affect any part of the GI tract, and there are two main types: ulcerative colitis and Crohn's disease.

Inflammation is present on multiple layers of the GI tract, like the esophagus, stomach, small intestine, and colon. It's more likely to develop between the ages of 15 and 30.

Diagnosing the condition involves blood or stool tests, biopsy, colonoscopy, or endoscopy.

Types:

With Crohn's disease, inflammation can happen anywhere in the GI tract. In cases of ulcerative colitis, the inflammation is limited to the large intestine (colon).

The symptoms of Crohn's disease and ulcerative colitis can vary widely. Some people experience mild symptoms. However, others experience severe symptoms that make their lives difficult. The severity of the symptoms will depend on the extent and length of the condition.

Ulcerative Colitis:

Ulcerative colitis causes inflammation and ulcers of the innermost lining of the large intestine. It usually develops in the rectum and may spread to the entire colon. There are several types of ulcerative colitis, depending on the area of the colon affected.

The most common symptoms include rectal bleeding or blood in stool, diarrhea, abdominal pain, weight loss, and fatigue. Ulcerative colitis can also cause joint pain and skin rashes.

Crohn's Disease:

Crohn's disease is a lifelong condition causing digestive tract inflammation. It generally affects the small intestine but can also harm other areas of the digestive tract in different people, including the mouth, stomach, and large intestine.

A person with Crohn's disease may have inflammation that affects the thickness of the intestinal wall, called transmural inflammation. This inflammation can lead to ulcers, infections, anal tears, and narrowing of the intestines. The healthy parts of the intestine overlap with inflamed areas, so the diagnosis and remedial approaches are tricky.

Causes:

The following are some potential causes of IBD:

Compromised immune system: A compromised immune system can lead to the body attacking itself. When this happens, the tissue lining the intestines can become inflamed and ulcerated.

Genes: Genes affect how our bodies respond to infection and injury. Genes may also influence how we react to certain foods or medicines. For example, if we have a family member diagnosed with IBD, there's a higher chance that we will develop it, too, since there's an inherited component.

Environmental triggers: Environmental factors play a role in IBD. Common factors are diet and stress. There are also air and water pollution, poor lifestyle choices that include smoking, lack of physical activity, and drugs or prescribed medicine like antibiotics.

Symptoms:

The symptoms of ulcerative colitis and Crohn's can be similar but vary from person to person.

They typically include:

- Persistent diarrhea
- Abdominal pain
- Bloody or mucous stools and rectal bleeding

- Fatigue
- Weight loss

Complications:

These are some potential complications of IBD:

Colon/Colorectal cancer: IBD can increase the risk of colon or colorectal cancer by as much as 20%, so it's vital to get regular screenings. The recommendation is to have one every three years starting at age 40.

Anal issues: Anal fissures and abscesses are common. The causes can include the inflammation of the rectum's lining or infected fecal material. These conditions may cause pain or bleeding during a bowel movement.

Anemia: People with IBD often experience anemia due to poor absorption of nutrients like B-12 and iron. In addition, there might be bleeding in the intestinal tract. This blood loss can result in anemia.

Kidney stones: In Crohn's disease, the intestine can't absorb fats properly, leading to an excess of a specific chemical in the kidney: oxalate, which can form kidney stones ("Cleveland Clinic," 2021).

Tears in the large intestine: These tears happen when inflammation causes the walls of the intestines to weaken and become damaged over time. These increase the risk of infection because bacteria can enter through these tears during bowel movements.

Malnutrition: Malnutrition is prevalent in IBD patients due to poor absorption, blood loss, and possible bacterial overgrowth.

Therapeutical Approach:

Although there's no cure for IBD, dietary changes will help manage the symptoms. The first step is to remove from the diet trigger foods like alcohol and caffeine; spicy, fried, and fatty foods; dairy products; carbonated drinks; fructose and other products with added sugar; raw and high-fiber foods such as fruits and vegetables; and nuts and legumes.

If you have this condition, focus on a diet rich in lean proteins such as poultry, fish, eggs, firm tofu, and kefir, as these can be tolerable.

Surprisingly, IBD patients do well when consuming refined starchy foods like pasta, oatmeal, rice, or bread made with white flour.

Cooking vegetables or fruits thoroughly, without seeds or skin, is recommended for plant-based foods. This process helps reduce the amount of (insoluble) fiber and will make these foods easier to digest. These food options include potatoes, carrots, and spinach. Avoiding large meals can also help.

To help soothe the inflammation associated with IBD, remedies with anti-inflammatory properties like Boswellia (frankincense), glucosamine, turmeric (curcumin), berberine, aloe vera, licorice, slippery elm, and wheatgrass juice should be considered.

Vitamin D3, iron, vitamin B12, and zinc will supplement the poor nutrient absorption from food. Omega-3 or fish oils will help in reducing inflammation.

Prebiotics (a type of fiber) and probiotics (friendly bacteria) are essential. Probiotics can help alleviate some of the symptoms as they help restore and balance microbiota. Prebiotics will support the growth of beneficial bacteria in the intestine.

Drinking water and consuming small meals throughout the day help keep digestion moving smoothly (Villines, 20218), particularly during flare-ups. Smaller meals are easier to digest and give the body time to absorb nutrients and control symptoms.

Stay hydrated as inflammation affects the colon mucosa and its ability to retain water; this can cause dehydration.

GERD

Gastroesophageal Reflux Disease (GERD) causes the muscle between the esophagus and stomach not to close adequately. This results in stomach acid frequently flowing back up and leading to irritation.

GERD can cause heartburn, regurgitation, hoarseness, difficulty swallowing, and chest pain. Transient acid refluxes can sometimes cause the symptoms. But, if experienced more than twice a week, it may be GERD.

Causes:

One cause of GERD is the abnormal relaxation or weakening of the muscles around the bottom of the esophagus. In turn, the valve between the esophagus and stomach weakens, allowing stomach acid to move up into the esophagus.

A considerable risk factor for GERD is obesity, as it puts extra pressure on the stomach and thus increases pressure on the lower esophageal sphincter. Other GERD risk factors include a hiatal hernia, pregnancy, and scleroderma. In a hiatal hernia, the stomach presses through the diaphragm into the chest cavity, potentially causing acid to move up the esophagus, leading to GERD symptoms. Pregnancy can also increase risk due to hormonal changes that cause lower esophageal sphincter relaxation (LES). Scleroderma is a condition that leads to the hardening of the skin and other organs in the body, including the esophagus ("Gastroesophageal Reflux," 2022). These factors may lead to heartburn or difficulty swallowing. Still, there are proponents that another risk factor is the presence of the H. Pylori bacteria, which can aggravate the condition.

The most common triggers or aggravating factors that can worsen symptoms are:

- Large meals or late eating
- Trigger foods such as those fried or high in fat
- Certain beverages like alcohol and caffeine
- Certain medications, such as aspirin

A doctor may diagnose the condition by performing an endoscopy or radiography.

Symptoms:

- Burning sensation in the chest, throat, or back that gets worse after eating or lying down
- Chest pain
- Regurgitation
- Difficulty swallowing
- Feeling like there's a lump in the throat
- Dry cough

Complications:

GERD can lead to several complications, including:

Esophagitis: This is a condition where the lining of the esophagus gets irritated and inflamed.

Esophageal cancer: A severe but rare form of cancer that begins in the esophagus lining, often due to damage from chronic acid reflux.

Narrowing of the esophagus: Potentially caused by scarred tissue due to chronic GERD.

Esophageal ulcers: Ulcers are sores that develop inside the esophagus and can cause bleeding, pain, difficulty swallowing, and cancer.

Therapeutic Approach:

There are several ways to address GERD and prevent its symptoms:

The best way to reduce symptoms is by avoiding foods that increase pressure in the upper abdomen, affect peristalsis, or slow down gastric emptying (food movement from the stomach to the intestine).

These foods include fatty or spicy foods, alcohol, carbonated beverages, citrus fruits, tomatoes, garlic, onion, and coffee.

Avoiding large meals that will put pressure on the stomach and focusing instead on consuming smaller meals throughout the day can bring relief.

Herbal remedies like licorice root, slippery elm, marshmallow, aloe vera, and chamomile will soothe and calm the stomach and esophagus.

These herbal remedies have been used for centuries for their soothing and restorative properties. Drinking diluted apple cider vinegar or water with lemon can also help to balance stomach acidity. Consuming fennel seeds before eating will aid in relaxing intestinal muscles. Ginger and turmeric are also known to help relieve symptoms of acid reflux. In addition, digestive enzymes can help in food breakdown to improve absorption, and hydrochloric acid can help restore the stomach's natural acidity.

Adding mastic gum, resin from a tree that has properties to relieve acid reflux and stomach ulcers, will help. It may contain antibacterial properties, so it can help fight H. Pylori bacteria if present.

As we've seen, all these digestive conditions are often related to microbiome imbalances and can lead to common symptoms or more dangerous complications. Removing triggering foods is often the first approach. The addition of supplements and other remedies will also have an impact on reducing symptoms.

5

IRRITABLE BOWEL SYNDROME (IBS)

Irritable Bowel Syndrome (IBS), like IBD, SIBO, Candidiasis, celiac disease, leaky gut, and GERD, is a common digestive disorder affecting about 15% of the US population and is associated with a microbiota imbalance. IBS affects the large and small intestines and is a chronic condition that needs management in the long term.

IBS has many possible symptoms, but pain, diarrhea, and constipation are the most common. The severity of these symptoms can vary. Some people may experience diarrhea and constipation at different times, while others might only experience one or the other.

IBS isn't considered a dangerous illness, and it's not life-threatening. However, it can be very debilitating because it affects the quality of life by limiting the ability to go out, work, or play sports due to pain and discomfort. Life can be a constant struggle when suffering from an IBS condition.

Just getting out of bed in the morning can be a struggle because of the fear that an episode or flare-up might occur at the most inconvenient moment. The symptoms can be more severe during these attacks and last hours or months.

There are ways to manage IBS and reduce the control it has in our lives. We can't control it, but there are steps to manage the symptoms. The first step is understanding what triggers it—and how it affects our bodies.

SYMPTOMS:

IBS symptoms can be embarrassing, especially when we don't understand why our bodies react like they do. Most people aren't bothered by the symptoms all the time; some only have symptoms once in a while, while others experience them often.

Abdominal pain related to bowel movements: Pain can be among the most common symptoms. This pain is usually felt in the lower abdomen and can worsen after eating and be relieved after a bowel movement. What causes these pains is believed to be poor signaling between the brain and the intestine.

Bloating: Bloating can result from increased gas production in the intestines due to the fermentation of undigested food particles in the colon, which causes gas.

Diarrhea, constipation, or both: Diarrhea can be caused by the intestinal muscles contracting faster than usual and matter moving through without allowing water to be absorbed. On the other hand, constipation can occur due to a slow motility process and a slow transit time that permits the colon to retain too much water from matter.

Excessive gas: It is often caused by the fermentation of undigested food particles in the large intestine. Also, food that moves too quickly through the digestive tract may result in trapped gas.

Feeling of incomplete evacuation: Also called tenesmus, this can occur when anal and pelvic muscles' coordination is impaired, causing incomplete bowel movements.

CAUSES:

It can be frustrating to deal with IBS symptoms because there's no apparent cause. The exact origin is unknown, but as we explored in earlier chapters, the brain and gut interact with each other to control digestive movements. This communication path may be abnormal or unbalanced in an IBS condition, leading to particular symptoms (Kennedy, 2014).

Muscle Contractions: The muscles in the intestines may contract too strongly or for too long, not strong enough, or for shorter periods. These abnormal processes can lead to symptoms and changes in the frequency of bowel movements.

Infections: An infection can be a precursor to IBS, too. Infections caused by bacteria, viruses, or parasites can lead to IBS. When there is an infection, the immune system sends white blood cells to the affected site. These cells release chemicals that can cause inflammation. The inflammation may, in turn, cause muscle spasms and cramps in the gastrointestinal tract, leading to abdominal pain and cramping. Diarrhea is also common when there's an infection because the body releases water into the colon to flush out the microorganism causing it.

Genetics and Environmental Factors: Although a prominent genetic component hasn't been identified as the cause of IBS, family history can be a significant risk factor. Relatives of IBS patients are most likely to develop the condition. However, environmental factors such as dietary habits can significantly affect whether a person develops the disorder.

Microbiota Imbalances: Another possible cause is an imbalance in gut microbiota—an overgrowth of certain bacteria types or an imbalance between good and bad bacteria. This imbalance can happen for many reasons, including poor eating habits, chronic stress, or the use of antibiotics.

It might not just be the presence or absence of particular microbes that cause problems but how the processes of these microorganisms affect each other. Some bacteria strains produce short-chain fatty acids, like butyrate, when they break down fiber. These compounds are essential for digestion and keeping the immune system strong. But too much may trigger symptoms. Even if these bacteria don't cause the issue, their processes are enough to cause digestive disturbances.

TYPES:

Two main IBS types are constipation (IBS-C) and diarrhea (IBS-D). Two other less common types are mixed bowel movement (IBS-M) and IBS-U or "unclassified," "unsubtyped," or "undefined." IBS-M manifests as periods of constipation alternating with periods of diarrhea. Painful cramping throughout the abdomen can be a symptom. People with IBS-M tend to have more overall symptoms than those diagnosed with either C or D alone. In IBS-U, symptoms of IBS don't fit into either the diarrhea or constipation category.

TRIGGERS:

Not knowing what sets off the symptoms of an IBS episode or flare-up can be frustrating. The specific triggers can be different for each person, and the only way to determine this is by keeping track of the foods or particular situations that occurred near the onset of the symptoms. Typical triggers include food and stress, but medications and hormones can also be culprits.

1) Food:

Although not the cause of IBS, food is a common offender, so much so that pain or other symptoms can worsen after eating certain things. Some may experience a sensitivity to any of the following:

High FODMAP (Fermentable, Oligosaccharides, Disaccharides, Monosaccharides, and Polyols):

High FODMAPs are fermentable sugars or carbohydrates commonly found in some grains, legumes, dairy, vegetables, and fruits. These foods can be hard to digest, and their absorption in the intestines is impaired. The undigested particles will ferment and produce excess water and gases, triggering the symptoms.

Fiber: Fiber is essential for optimal digestive health. However, too much or too little or the type of fiber consumed can trigger reactions. Insoluble fiber, which moves quickly through the intestines and is commonly found in leafy greens, seeds, legumes, and nuts, can negatively impact those who suffer from IBS-D, the diarrhea type. Most foods considered high in FODMAPs have fiber.

Caffeinated beverages: Although coffee is considered low in FODMAPs, it contains other compounds that can speed up motility in the intestines, thus causing more diarrhea.

Chocolate: Due to its caffeine content and being high in fats, it can activate IBS responses. The good news is that chocolate, especially in its dark form or cacao powder, is considered low in FODMAPs and is safe to eat in small quantities.

Alcohol: There are some alcoholic drinks considered low in FODMAPs, but the recommendation is to consume them in moderation. Alcohol irritates the intestines and affects the digestion of carbohydrates, resulting in IBS symptoms.

Fatty foods: Fatty foods often worsen people's diarrhea because they slow digestion and cause intestinal gas build-up.

Highly processed foods: Processed foods often include food coloring, additives, sweeteners, and other ingredients that can be high in FODMAPs or other substances to which we can be sensitive, thus setting off IBS reactions.

2) Stress:

Stress is another significant factor related to IBS. Just like food, stress isn't considered the cause, but when present, the symptoms can worsen. Stress often causes overactivity in the gut, and one possible reason is the excess of cortisol, a hormone released during stressful situations.

Cortisol triggers multiple reactions in the body, including those that affect digestion. These reactions affect the colon and the microbiota balance. An imbalanced microbiota will negatively influence the processing of stress responses and how the brain communicates with the gut (Sugaya et al., 2015).

RISK FACTORS:

IBS is most common among people younger than age 50, particularly in women. It's not clear whether any lifestyle choices affect this.

Some hormone therapies specific to women affect IBS. Estrogen therapy for menopause, birth control pills, or intrauterine devices (IUDs) can cause bowel irritation. Sex hormones, particularly estrogen, affect "visceral sensitivity, motility, permeability, and immune activation of intestinal mucosa" (Mulak et al., 2014). Estrogen changes the normal function of the bowels as it may worsen symptoms in some people, but in others, it relieves them.

A history of physical or mental abuse is also a risk factor. Emotional or sexual abuse can increase the risk of IBS. This trauma and the stress associated can aggravate and worsen symptoms (Sansone et al., 2015).

Certain medications may cause responses similar to IBS. These medications include antibiotics and nonsteroidal anti-inflammatory drugs (NSAIDs), generally used as pain relievers, antidepressants, or antacids.

DIAGNOSIS:

IBS has no specific test or lab that confirms its presence. Instead, doctors diagnose it based on medical history and physical exams. They'll also consider other conditions that could be very similar to or be related to IBS.

To diagnose it, your doctor will review symptoms and may ask about the following:

- Bowel habits and how often they occur
- Symptoms related to abdominal pain
- Other problems associated with digestion, such as nausea and vomiting
- They may also suggest the following:

- o Lactose intolerance test to rule out lactose sensitivity
- o Breath test to rule out SIBO
- o Stool test to rule out bacteria or parasite presence

COMPLICATIONS:

There aren't many IBS complications. Usually, this chronic condition stays with the patient for a long time and can sometimes lead to:

Migraines/headaches: Headaches are one of the most typical complications related to IBS. Some of us may have migraine headaches unrelated to IBS, potentially triggered by stress or certain foods. There seems to be a genetic link between these two conditions, and people with IBS are twice as likely to suffer from migraines. Serotonin and brain-gut axis processes are parts of this correlation.

Fibromyalgia: Fibromyalgia is another condition linked to IBS. Fibromyalgia causes muscle pain throughout the body that worsens with inactivity and improves with exercise. People with fibromyalgia also experience fatigue and muscle tenderness when touched (called tender points). Studies indicate that a high number of IBS patients also experience fibromyalgia. Both conditions tend to cause a higher pain sensitivity (Yang et al., 2020).

Sleep problems: Most people with IBS have difficulty sleeping. Sleep deprivation can worsen other symptoms, such as constipation and abdominal pain. Research also indicates a link between IBS, depression, and anxiety disorders.

Chronic pelvic pain (CPP): This pain can last more than six months and affects daily activities and quality of life. CPP is associated with IBS in up to 50% of cases and occurs more frequently in women than men. Chronic pelvic pain may be caused especially by IBS-C. This type of IBS puts more pressure on the lower muscles and bones, so CPP is likely to develop (Choung et al., 2010).

Interstitial cystitis. This chronic bladder condition involves painful episodes occurring at night or early morning. What causes interstitial cystitis is unclear, but it may have an autoimmune component. Interstitial cystitis is also a condition that IBS patients often suffer from.

Chronic fatigue syndrome (CFS). Persistent fatigue is a condition that doesn't improve with rest and worsens after physical or mental exertion. People with IBS may also experience CFS, although the cause is unknown.

IBS AND WOMEN:

Research indicates that IBS tends to be a more common disorder among women (Kim et al., 2018). A possible reason is that women have a slower gastrointestinal transit time than men. This slower motility can worsen symptoms because food stays in the colon longer, giving bacteria more time to produce gas and other substances that cause cramping and constipation, for example.

Hormonal changes are also a factor. The effects hormones have on IBS are so significant that the symptoms are often severe during a woman's menstrual cycle and postovulatory and premenstrual phases. These are the times when the hormones estrogen and progesterone increase. The increased levels can result in mood swings. Or it could be hormones causing both mood swings and bowel irritations. Women with painful periods or irregular cycles could be at increased risk for developing IBS.

Often, the symptoms of IBS and gynecological conditions are similar. According to research, around 50% of the patients who reported pain in the lower abdomen suffer from IBS, a non-gynecological disorder ("Women and Irritable Bowel Syndrome," 2010). Since they only experienced pain and no significant bowel issues, it was assumed the pain was related to hormones. While in a way it was, the disease was quite different than it appeared.

Far too often, the diseases themselves are interconnected. Studies indicate that people suffering from IBS may also have endometriosis at some point, and women with this condition are twice as likely to develop IBS. They also go through a higher hysterectomy rate than most ("Women and Irritable Bowel Syndrome," 2010).

THERAPEUTIC APPROACH:

Despite having no treatment, several approaches, such as diet, stress-relieving techniques, supplementation, and lifestyle changes, will help manage IBS symptoms.

Diet is essential in mitigating symptoms because it's beneficial in modifying the gut microbiome and reducing trigger foods like those that ferment and produce gas, pain, bloating, diarrhea, or constipation. A heavily recommended approach is the low FODMAP diet.

In the following chapters, we'll explore this approach and the potential benefits of adapting popular diets into our lifestyles to promote digestive health. Moreover, supplements, herbal remedies, stress-relieving practices, and other techniques can help manage symptoms.

————————

In summary, although not considered a serious health condition, IBS can impact the quality of life and is closely related to female hormonal issues. As well as stress, fermentable carbohydrates tend to trigger symptoms. Therefore, making dietary changes and focusing on a low FODMAP approach will likely help improve the condition.

6

EMBRACING THE LOW FODMAP AND NATURAL HOLISTIC APPROACH

As mentioned previously, medically speaking, there's no treatment for IBS. In cases of diarrhea, sometimes doctors may prescribe antibiotics if determined the cause is a bacterial infection. In most cases, IBS doesn't need any medical treatment at all.

The typical approach to address IBS is making lifestyle modifications. Often, and unsurprisingly, the food we eat worsens our symptoms. So, changing our eating habits can be part of the restorative approach, even if the food doesn't cause the problem.

One of the specialized diets nutritionists have been recommending is the Low FODMAP.

WHAT'S FODMAP?

FODMAP (Fermentable Oligosaccharides, Disaccharides, Monosaccharides, and Polyols) are carbohydrates (sugars, fiber, or starches) commonly found in fruits, vegetables, grains, legumes, and dairy ("FODMAP food list," 2019). Poor absorption of these carbohydrates can occur in the small intestine. This process can cause fermentation, increased gas production, bloating, or abdominal distension.

FODMAP ORIGINS

In the early 2000s, researchers at Monash University in Australia noticed that certain foods sparked symptoms in some people, causing intestinal conditions, and reducing the intake of these foods would help alleviate IBS symptoms. This approach has shown success, and studies indicate a reduction of symptoms in more than 80% of patients who follow this way of eating (Gearry et al., 2016).

TYPES OF FODMAP FOODS

Let's take a look at the four types of carbohydrates (saccharides) categorized in FODMAPs:

Oligosaccharides *(Fructans in grains and vegetables, galactans in legumes)*:

Oligosaccharides are carbohydrates with many smaller molecules or monosaccharides (simple sugar particles). Oligosaccharides are classified as fructans or fructo-oligosaccharides (FOS) and galactans or galacto-oligosaccharides (GOS). Enzymes in our digestive tract don't digest these sugars, so they pass through us undigested to the large intestine. There, fermentation is likely, leading to digestive symptoms.

These are examples of foods high in oligosaccharides:

Fructans:

Grains: Barley, Bran, cous cous, farro, gnocchi, rye, semolina, spelt and wheat
Nuts/seeds: Cashews and pistachios
Vegetables: Artichokes, asparagus, broccoli, brussels sprouts, cabbage, garlic, leek, okra, onions, peas and shallots
Fruits:Grapefruit, persimmon, pomegranate, ripe bananas, and watermelon

Galactans:

Legumes:Beans, chickpeas, lentils, split peas and soybeans

Disaccharides (*Lactose in dairy, sucrose in fruits)*:

Disaccharides are formed by combining two monosaccharides or simple sugars. There are many types, but the most common disaccharides are lactose in milk and its derivatives and sucrose in fruits. Because these sugars are poorly absorbed, their consumption can cause bloating and gas when fermented by bacteria in the large intestine.

These are other examples of Disaccharides:

Sucrose and Maltose: Apricots, peaches, fruit drinks, and table sugar
Lactose: Dairy: buttermilk, cream cheese, custard, ice cream, milk (cow, sheep and goat), ricotta cheese, sour cream, and yogurt

Monosaccharides *(Fructose and glucose in fruits and sweeteners)*:

Monosaccharides are sugars in fruits and other sweeteners. They're the simplest form of carbohydrates or the most basic type of sugars; two types are glucose and fructose. Glucose in the small intestine often draws water, causing the intestine to expand. Bloating and gas result when fermentation in the large intestine occurs. Fructose can be poorly absorbed, but in small quantities, there's a better chance of increased absorption; in large amounts, however, the unabsorbed portions will cause bloating and gas when fermented in the large intestine.

These are some common monosaccharide foods:

> **Fruits**: Apples, dry fruits, mangoes, pears, cherries, and cranberries
> **Sweeteners**: Agave, corn syrup, honey, malt and molasses

Polyols *(sweeteners, fruits, and vegetables)*:

Polyols are sugar alcohols in fruits and artificial sweeteners like sorbitol, xylitol, and maltitol. Vegetables like cauliflower, mushrooms, and stone fruits like peaches and plums contain this type of sugar. Polyols are commonly used as food additives because they're low in calories. Different foods and beverages may contain polyols, including chewing gum, hard candy, toothpaste, and mouthwash.

Polyols can cause gastrointestinal symptoms if consumed in large quantities. Like the other carbohydrates identified in FODMAPs, they're poorly absorbed, draw water into the intestine, and ferment. Due to their laxative effects, foods containing polyols can cause diarrhea.

Examples of foods that contain polyols are:

Fruits: Blackberries, figs, lychees, nectarines, peaches, and plums
Sweeteners: Maltitol, mannitol, sorbitol, and xylitol
Vegetables: Cauliflower and mushrooms

FERMENTED AND FERMENTABLE FOODS

Fermentation is a conventional method to preserve food and improve its taste. However, "fermented" and "fermentable" foods are different. Fermented foods have already been semi-digested or broken down by bacteria. These foods, like yogurt or sauerkraut, can benefit the gut bacteria when consumed in moderation.

Fermentable foods, on the other hand, can be fermented or are usually fermented after we eat them, potentially in the intestines. The colon or large intestine mainly acts as a reservoir of bacteria, refines digestion, and aids in processing carbohydrates through fermentation.

Fermentable carbohydrates move slowly through the intestine. Enzymes don't break them down in the small intestine and pass into the colon to be digested by bacteria. The extra water in the small intestine provides a favorable environment for fermentation by bacteria, and gas results as a by-product. This process can cause bloating and constipation as well.

FODMAPS AND GLUTEN:

Fermentable carbohydrates or FODMAPs aren't the same as gluten-containing foods. FODMAPs are carbohydrate compounds, and gluten is a protein in wheat, barley, and rye; interestingly, these grains are also considered high in FODMAPs. Gluten to celiac patients will cause digestive symptoms similar to those experienced in IBS, like abdominal pain, bloating, diarrhea, constipation, and gas. While fermentable carbohydrates in the intestine cause excess water and fermentation, gluten damages the villi or hairs covering the walls of the intestines.

SUGAR LEVELS AND INTENSITY OF SYMPTOMS

FODMAP foods fall into three categories based on their impact on the digestive system.

High-FODMAP foods contain the highest fermentable sugar levels and can cause the most digestive distress. This category includes legumes, asparagus, crucifers like broccoli, cabbage, and cauliflower, alliums such as garlic and onions, dairy, fruits, and grains like wheat, barley, and rye. These foods aggravate IBS symptoms and should be avoided or restricted for some time.

Moderate-FODMAP foods can cause mild symptoms. These should be consumed in small amounts, and then you can assess the reaction to determine if you need to avoid them for extended periods. These include avocado, bell peppers, butternut squash, celery, sweet potato, pumpkin, pomegranates, beets, and grapefruit.

Low-FODMAP foods cause little or no symptoms in people with IBS because these are low in fermentable sugars. Because sugars are only found in plant-based foods, unprocessed animal products, except for dairy, are free of FODMAPs, mainly if they're grass-fed. In this category, we can find red meats, poultry, eggs, fish, and other seafood.

These are other samples of low FODMAP foods:

Dairy:
Cheeses: brie, cheddar, cottage, feta, mozzarella, parmesan and Swiss
Others: butter and lactose-free milk and yogurt
Fruits: Blue berries, cantaloupes, grapes, honey dew, kiwi, most citrus fruits, papaya, passion fruit, pineapple, strawberry and unripe bananas
Vegetables: Arugula, bean sprouts, Bok choy, carrots, chives, collar greens, cucumbers, eggplants, fennel, kale, lettuce, olives, parsnips, spinach, tomatoes, turnips and zucchini
Protein: Eggs, firm tofu, tempeh, unprocessed meats
Nuts: Almonds, Brazilian nuts, chestnuts, hazelnuts, macadamia nuts, peanuts, pecans, pine nuts and walnuts
Seeds: Chia, Flax, hemp, poppy, pumpkin, sesame and sunflower
Grains: Buckwheat, millet, oat bran, oats, quinoa and rice
Starchy Vegetables: Corn, plantains, potatoes, squash, yam and yuca/cassava
Sweeteners: Aspartame, saccharine, stevia, sucralose

HOW DOES THE FODMAP APPROACH WORK?

The basis for this diet is to temporarily avoid foods high in FODMAP and focus instead on consuming low FODMAP foods. This elimination aims to help the gut bacteria get into better balance and eventually digest these foods more effectively. If necessary, the diet can be continued indefinitely until symptoms are alleviated or one has had adequate time to adapt to the new eating pattern.

The diet should be easy to follow, but working with a dietitian or gastroenterologist may be more effective as a professional can help tailor this approach to the individual needs.

PHASES OF THE FODMAP DIET

The FODMAP approach has three phases:

The elimination phase: High FODMAPs are eliminated for 2-6 weeks in the initial step. During this phase, foods to avoid are legumes, asparagus, artichokes, crucifers that include cauliflower, alliums such as garlic and onions, dairy, fruits like apples and peaches, and grains like wheat, barley, and rye. Instead, focus on consuming low or free food versions such as proteins, leafy greens, seeds, and some fruits and nuts (refer in sections above for a list of high and low FODMAP foods).

The reintroduction phase: The elimination phase is followed by reintroducing trigger foods individually and observing their effects. The reintroduction/rechallenge phase can last up to eight weeks. During this time, the objective is to add foods high in FODMAPs into the diet one at a time and to monitor how the body reacts and the symptoms that follow. It's also essential to determine the amount of food to consume and the order to add them back into the diet. If the symptoms persist, that food is potentially problematic and should be avoided longer. During this phase, a suggestion is to take a break between the reintroduction of each food to determine the effect of each.

The maintenance or personalization phase: Once the foods that affect the digestive symptoms are recognized, these are to be consumed only in moderation. This phase aims to tailor the diet to what works for each individual, avoid the foods that still cause issues, and consume tolerable foods.

DOES THE LOW FODMAP APPROACH WORK?

This diet has been trendy lately. But what are the downsides or drawbacks?

Well, there are a few. First, not everyone who follows this dietary approach sees improvements. About one in four people don't see any progression at all. Second, as this diet is restrictive and limits foods rich in nutrients such as legumes, vegetables, and fruits (especially for those who follow it for a long time), there's a risk of nutritional deficiencies, impacting our overall health. Thirdly, many people find that following this diet potentially triggers eating disorders—especially when combined with other restrictive diets like veganism or vegetarianism. If continued for extended periods, it can result in an imbalance of gut microbiota due to the reduction in fiber, which is beneficial for gut health. It can also be challenging to stick with because our diet consists of more than simple ingredients. Our diet includes restaurant foods, takeout, candies, desserts, etc. So, we aren't necessarily aware of what goes into our food all the time.

Even so, it's always worth giving it a try since, for many, it has been an absolute blessing!

SUPPLEMENTATION

Undoubtedly, a change in diet is the most critical factor for managing symptoms of IBS and other gastrointestinal problems. However, supplementation with herbal and natural remedies can act wonderfully in relieving symptoms.

Herbal remedies like aloe vera, slippery elm, ginger, turmeric, artichoke leaf extract, and peppermint may relieve symptoms without causing side effects.

- Peppermint can help keep the intestines moving smoothly and support the immune system to stay strong.
- Aloe vera and slippery elm have anti-inflammatory properties and may help relieve constipation and soothe the digestive tract.
- Ginger has pain relief properties that can improve bowel movements and calm nausea.
- Turmeric helps reduce inflammation and improve gut motility.

- Chamomile tea and artichoke leaf extract may help
  soothe an irritated digestive tract and ease symptoms of
  diarrhea and constipation.

In Ayurvedic medicine, a holistic approach, Triphala is a traditional remedy for gastrointestinal disorders. It has cleansing and detoxing properties and can help with abdominal pain, bloating, and constipation. Amalaki fruit is another Ayurvedic remedy that can mitigate constipation due to its laxative effects.

Probiotics are live microorganisms or good bacteria that promote digestive health. Prebiotics is a dietary fiber that can't be digested but, in the large intestine, serves as a food source for bacteria. Digestive enzymes are proteins that help break down food and convert it into particles easily absorbed in the intestine. Probiotics, prebiotics, and digestive enzymes are all essential to a comprehensive relief plan for IBS.

All vitamins are essential to supplement our diet to prevent nutritional deficiencies. Often, when we suffer from IBS, we're deficient in vitamin D. This vitamin helps regulate inflammation in the body and can help manage symptoms of IBS. It's also crucial for absorbing other nutrients and supports immunity. Vitamin B6 and B12 are also needed. Vitamin B6 is associated with serotonin metabolism and how the nervous system relates to gastrointestinal functions. B12 also affects how nerve signals occur between the brain and the gut.

Amino acids, molecules that build proteins, can play a role in preventing and remediating inflammation in the gut and restoring the intestinal barrier. An essential amino acid is L-glutamine, which can help prevent infection and inflammation of the intestine's mucous membrane. It also plays a role in maintaining the balance of microbiota. Glutathione (a molecule of three amino acids) is a powerful antioxidant that can protect against inflammation inside the digestive tract.

LIFESTYLE CHANGES

Dietary changes and supplementation are crucial for managing IBS symptoms. But sometimes, just making small lifestyle changes can have a positive outcome.

The consumption of smaller meals throughout the day will help us balance out the digestive system, and it will also help to stave off hunger pangs.

Another good practice is to cook meals at home. We can control the quantity and types of ingredients we use and what goes into our bodies if we're involved in preparing our food.

Keeping a diary will help us track what we eat and the associated symptoms.

Chewing food thoroughly and slowly eating is also a smart idea. Chewing triggers signals sent to the stomach to release digestive enzymes and stomach acid needed for proper digestion. Chewing food all the way through ensures foods have been broken down into digestible pieces to prevent large particles from entering the intestines and setting off reactions. Eating slowly will help us relax, and in a relaxed state, digestion is enhanced.

To wrap up this chapter, FODMAP is a common food approach for IBS and other digestive conditions where inflammation, gas, constipation, and diarrhea are common symptoms. Learning how fermentable foods can be adapted to our diet and adding supplements and other techniques can bring us relief.

7

ALTERNATIVE DIETS AND IMPLICATIONS FOR DIGESTIVE WELLNESS

While the FODMAP approach remains relevant for managing IBS, SIBO, and other digestive disorders, understanding other diets can help us adapt them to our dietary lifestyles. In addition, because the FODMAP approach may only work for some, we need to learn how to incorporate foods or diets into our daily regimen.

Many popular diets have the goal of improving our health. The bad news is that, in general, those diets may not necessarily help improve our specific digestive disorders. So, finding an approach that works for us can be tricky if we suffer from gastrointestinal conditions. Some of us IBS sufferers must avoid certain foods, while others can consume them in moderation. Either way, there's no standard diet that works for everyone. But, with the proper knowledge, we can learn how to incorporate and use food combinations that benefit us.

Here are the most popular diets and the foods they cover.

KETO

A ketogenic (keto) diet is characterized by restricting the consumption of carbohydrates and increasing the intake of fats and proteins. Ketone substances are produced in our bodies when carbohydrate consumption is limited, and proteins and fats are the primary sources of calories. Our body can use ketones as the energy source instead of glucose produced when we consume carbohydrates.

Keto foods

What foods are allowed on a keto diet?

- Healthy fats: nuts and seeds, butter, avocado, MCT, and olive oil
- Proteins: poultry, red meats, eggs, fish, and other seafood and organ meats
- Fruits low in sugar: citrus and berries
- Vegetables low in starches: like leafy greens, tomatoes, and eggplants
- Dairy products: cheese, kefir, and yogurt

Origins of the keto diet

The keto diet was developed to help treat seizures in children with epilepsy (Wheless, 2008). This eating method forces our body to use fats rather than carbohydrates as a source of energy. Typically, our body metabolizes carbohydrates into glucose, which is transported around the body and is particularly important for fueling physical activity. However, if carbohydrate consumption is limited, the liver transforms fat into fatty acids and ketone substances; the presence of ketones in our blood is known as ketosis. The ketone bodies are taken to the brain, replacing glucose as an energy source.

Although keto is now commonly used for weight loss, it has also shown potential benefits in improving the symptoms of metabolic syndrome—a collection of health conditions that affect blood sugar and heart health—in adults.

For an IBS condition, some evidence suggests it can help manage symptoms (Gigante et al., 2021). Some people find that reducing their intake of carbohydrates can help ease their symptoms. The reason for this improvement is probably the elimination of many high-FODMAP foods like grains and legumes.

Promising research shows that following the keto approach can help reduce bowel inflammation. According to a study, ketone bodies have anti-inflammatory effects through various mechanisms, including decreasing intestinal Th17 cells. These cells are part of an immune response that causes inflammation and can lead to immune diseases (Ang et al.,2020).

While this diet can be healthy, it's only for some or not for the long term. Some people may experience fatigue, headaches, constipation, and nausea when starting the plan.

Our kidneys and liver may become overloaded because of the high fat and protein content, increasing the risk to these organs. The excess acid produced from the digestion of protein sources can cause a decrease in blood pH. In the long term, high levels of acidity can cause the formation of kidney stones; it can also cause a reduction in the density of bone minerals and loss of muscle mass, as well as an increase in the risk of chronic diseases like hypertension (Carnauba et al., 2017).

A keto diet may cause an increase in leaky gut syndrome and abdominal pain. One possible reason is the consumption of a high-fat diet, which can impair genetic components that maintain the integrity of the intestinal lining ("What Impact," 2020).

Not to mention, the diet can be restrictive, which means missing out on some essential nutrients. For example, a deficiency might develop in vitamins and minerals like selenium, magnesium, potassium, and B9 (folate), commonly found in plant-based foods.

In addition, when we eat a lot of animal products, getting enough fiber is challenging. This lack of fiber can negatively impact our gut microbiome and lead to constipation and other bowel problems.

Despite the potential to negatively impact our digestion, we can modify the ketogenic diet to meet our needs. Many food fiber sources are still permitted. We can focus on healthy proteins, leafy greens, and healthy fats. In addition, supplementing with fiber or prebiotics and including enough probiotics can help balance our microbiome. Furthermore, following this approach for a shorter time, typically up to six months, is generally recommended to minimize adverse effects.

PALEO

The paleo diet takes us back to the prehistoric era, over two million years ago when humans lived as hunters and gatherers. Often called the caveman diet, this approach was introduced by Dr. Walter L. Voegtlin in 1975 but made popular in 2002 by Dr. Loren Cordain, believed to be the founder of the Paleo Movement.

The paleo diet advocates that we should eat what our ancestors ate before agriculture about 10,000 years ago because our bodies haven't evolved much since then.

The paleo diet consists of:

- Lean meats, fish and other seafood, eggs, vegetables, fruits, and nuts
- Seeds are optional or allowed in small quantities or only in some varieties
- Dairy is often avoided if following the diet in its strictest form
- Grains, refined sugar, processed foods, and legumes are also avoided

Paleo and keto diets are very similar. However, the ketogenic approach focuses on reducing carbohydrates, so starchy vegetables, sweeteners, and fruits are restricted. The paleo diet recommends removing foods not part of the diet in the hunter and gathering age, such as grains, legumes, and processed foods, which tend to cause inflammation in our bodies.

The benefit of paleo is that it's low in carbohydrates and can lower blood pressure, improve insulin sensitivity, and help with weight loss. This diet also helps improve digestive health by eliminating foods that may cause inflammation; these foods are often considered high in FODMAPs. This elimination can be beneficial if we suffer from IBS, IBD, SIBO, and gluten or lactose sensitivities. Limiting processed foods with added chemicals that stimulate chronic inflammation in the GI tract is also a potential advantage of the paleo diet.

Although it can offer many benefits for our health, we should only follow this diet for a short time, as it has some adverse effects on digestive health in the long term, including altering the microbial composition of the intestine and causing our microbiome to lose key components (Genoni et al., 2019).

VEGAN AND VEGETARIAN

The vegan or vegetarian approach is a lifestyle that focuses on adhering to a plant-based diet.

A vegan diet includes eating vegetables and fruits, nuts/seeds, grains, and legumes; no animal products are allowed. Strict vegans also avoid using products made from animals, such as leather shoes or silk clothing.

Vegetarians, on the other hand, in addition to plant-based food, often consume eggs and dairy products. Some vegetarians may consume poultry, fish, or both. Terms such as ovolactovegetarians (consume eggs and dairy), pescatarians (consume fish), or pollotarians (consume poultry) are used to describe vegetarians whose diets include non-plant-based foods.

There are several reasons people adopt a vegan or vegetarian lifestyle. For some people, it's for ethical reasons because they may think that eating animal products is cruel and unnecessary. Others may do it because they believe plants are better for the environment than animals. Another reason may be that plant-based diets are healthier for our bodies. Whatever the reason, vegetarianism is a typical diet in many cultures and has been around for thousands of years. These diets have been known in the West for several decades, and the benefits are well documented.

A well-balanced vegan or vegetarian diet can be healthy and delicious. It may reduce the chance of heart disease and help with losing weight. Compared to a standard American diet, a well-planned vegetarian or vegan diet provides nutrients, fiber, and antioxidants, which will help keep blood sugar under control and reduce inflammation. Fiber is fantastic for promoting the growth of lactic acid bacteria, which is essential for our health.

Like fiber, polyphenols in plant-based food also increase Bifidobacterium and Lactobacillus species, providing anti-pathogenic and anti-inflammatory effects. These can also help with cardiovascular protection. The high consumption of vegetarian foods also encourages SCFA (short-chain fatty acid) production.

According to scientists, the health effects of SCFA include "improved immunity against pathogens, blood-brain barrier integrity, provision of energy substrates, and regulation of critical functions of the intestine." (Tomova et al., 2019)

Nevertheless, a plant-based approach, while providing excellent benefits for our health, can increase digestive symptoms, possibly caused by the high levels of foods high in fermentable sugars such as grains, fruits, and legumes, including soy products, which is unfortunate because soy contains a lot of protein. Because most plant-based protein sources fall under high FODMAPs, vegetarians and vegans have limited protein options.

A strictly plant-based diet may lack several nutritional components, including vitamin B12, vitamin D, calcium, zinc, magnesium, and iron. Missing one of these nutrients can lead to anemia, slow recovery, and an impact on hormones.

MEDITERRANEAN

The Mediterranean diet has been popular in the Mediterranean region for thousands of years. It's similar to modern-day diets and emphasizes whole grains, legumes, fruit, vegetables, nuts, seeds, olive oil, and poultry; moderate fish consumption, unprocessed cheese, and yogurt are allowed. Red meat is avoided or limited to minimal amounts. The consumption of wine is optional but recommended in moderate amounts. ("Cleveland Clinic," 2022).

The Mediterranean diet is an excellent way to stay healthy because it includes fiber-rich foods; this increases microbiota diversity and promotes gut homeostasis and the balance of good and bad bacteria in the digestive tract.

Olive oil, prevalent in this diet, is rich in polyphenol antioxidants, which have anti-inflammatory and antimicrobial properties.

The properties of polyphenols and other nutrients in typical Mediterranean diet foods can help reduce digestive symptoms common in IBS conditions, like bloating and abdominal pain, without causing adverse effects on bowels like those observed with other fiber supplements or foods. These positive effects may be possible because of the production of short-chain fatty acids (SCFA) from complex and insoluble fiber, which are known to protect against intestinal diseases (Nagpal et al., 2019).

But, the benefits of the Mediterranean diet go beyond digestion. It also helps prevent inflammatory diseases and allergies. It can support the reduction of obesity, diabetes, cardiovascular disease, bowel disease, and cancer (Mentella et al., 2019).

However, because the diet includes many high-FODMAP foods such as whole grains, legumes, and fruits, it should be customized for proper digestive health. Our focus should be on consuming a variety of foods low in FODMAPs, like unprocessed meats, poultry, eggs, fish and vegetables, and fruits. The consumption of legumes like chickpeas, nuts, seeds, grains, and high FODMAP vegetables and fruits should be avoided or limited based on our symptoms.

The Mediterranean diet can benefit our digestive and overall health if adjusted accordingly.

INTERMITTENT FASTING

There are many different approaches to dieting. Some of us may eat very little, and others may choose to eat specific foods or follow a particular diet. One approach that's become very common in recent years is intermittent fasting or "IF."

Intermittent fasting comprises alternating between periods of eating and fasting. One of the most common forms is the 16:8 method: fasting for 16 hours each day and then limiting eating to an eight-hour window. For example, the last meal of the day is at 5 PM, and the first meal the following day is at 9 AM.

Other forms include alternate-day fasting (ADF) and 5:2 fasting or fasting two days a week.

Alternate day fasting (ADF) is an eating pattern involving eating one day and then fasting on the second. ADF isn't recommended for beginners since it can be hard to stick to this kind of pattern long term.

In a 5:2 method, the focus is to eat as you usually do for five days and fast for two days. Fasting doesn't need to occur on consecutive days; the point is to eat less food than usual on the two fasting days. The most common strategy is to eat less than one-third of the calories usually consumed. This approach can help reduce obesity risk factors like blood pressure and cholesterol ("World-First Study," 2018).

Although the effects of intermittent fasting are still being researched, results so far are promising. The positive is that it increases metabolism and improves overall gastrointestinal health. During fasting, the gut rests and recovers from digestion, which allows gut cleansing mechanisms to occur. These mechanisms remove old food particles and microbes that can trigger IBS symptoms. The extra space in our digestive tract also helps improve motility, which allows food to move through more efficiently than it would if we were eating all the time. Improved motility prevents excess fermentation of food and reduces the occurrence of SIBO, both of which are connected to IBS symptoms.

Intermittent fasting improves the gut microbiome by increasing beneficial bacteria while decreasing pathogenic bacteria. Intermittent fasting causes considerable changes in the gut microbiome and increases butyric acid-producing bacteria. This improved microbiota diversity can also positively affect insulin sensitivity (Su et al., 2021).

Think of fasting as a long, soothing bath for the intestines. Whether therapeutically or as a way to kickstart weight loss, it's one of the easiest and most effective ways to detoxify our body. During fasting, our body switches to autophagy, where damaged cells are destroyed and their components recycled into new cells. Also, proteins that help to prevent misfolding (an abnormal process) that may lead to cancer or other diseases are more receptive during fasting (Antunes et al., 2018).

Intermittent fasting also helps reset our inner clock or circadian rhythm, a 24-hour cycle regulating sleeping and waking. In a study, those who participated in intermittent fasting woke up less during the night. Hence, they had a more restful sleep ("The Benefits of," 2021).

Intermittent fasting is correlated with a healthy lifestyle. It isn't a restrictive diet but is easily adapted as a way of life. Implemented once or twice a week, it can allow our bodies to rest and our digestive system to clean itself and recover.

Despite its health benefits, caution should be observed during pregnancy or if suffering from an eating disorder. Similarly, practice with care if you have diabetes since sugar levels fluctuate during fasting.

LECTINS, GLUTEN, SOY, NIGHTSHADES, DAIRY, AND HISTAMINES

Although most natural foods are considered healthy and nutritious, some can cause an immunological response. Even if we aren't allergic, we can benefit from excluding certain foods from our diets, at least for some time. As we've explored in previous chapters, avoiding particular foods is especially important if we suffer digestive problems, hormonal imbalances, or other chronic conditions. When we suspect that we're negatively reacting to a food, a comprehensive stool or blood test or sensitivity analysis can help us to determine what's going on more precisely.

Why do certain foods trigger reactions in our bodies? Like high FODMAP foods that cause digestive symptoms, because particles tend to ferment in the intestine, other foods also contain compounds that can affect our health. Lectins, gluten, soy, dairy, and alkaloids are some examples.

Lectins

Lectins are a type of protein or glycoprotein found in plants. They have properties that allow them to attach to the cell surfaces of sugar molecules in our bodies. These properties can result in agglutination or the clumping of cells, triggering an immune response resulting in inflammation and consequently causing autoimmune disorders.

Whole grains, legumes, and peanuts are considered high in lectins. Seeds and the outer layer of vegetables, such as tomatoes and potatoes, and nuts like almonds and cashews are typical foods high in lectins. The same is true for processed products made with lectin-containing components. Lectins can be present in animal products; when poultry, pigs, and cows are fed grains or other similar foods, their eggs, milk, and meat may contain lectin. Products from pasture-raised animals or animals not fed grains are considered free or have low levels of lectins.

Although research is limited on the long-term effect of lectins, these substances are said to impact our bodies.

Lectins resist being broken down by enzymes, which can upset our digestion. If we suffer from a digestive condition like IBS, we could be more likely to react to these substances and experience typical symptoms. In extreme cases, lectins can also cause anaphylaxis (a severe allergic reaction) as these proteins can attach to cells lining the digestive tract, disrupting the breakdown and absorption of nutrients and affecting microbiota balance.

However, lectins can offer health benefits. They can slow carbohydrate digestion and absorption, preventing the sudden rise of glucose and keeping blood sugar levels regulated. Lectins act as antioxidants that protect cells from free radicals. Some of these types can have anti-tumor and antibacterial capabilities due to their binding properties to specific sugars on the surface of harmful microorganisms and malignant cells found in some cancers ("Lectins," 2019). Lectins may also have a role in enzyme and bile production and in stimulating gut motility that aids in food movement along the GI tract.

If we aren't affected negatively by lectin-containing foods, we have no reason to avoid them. As long as lectin-containing foods are prepared the right way, the negative effect of these proteins is reduced ("Lectins," 2019). Heat is known to break these particles down, so cooking beans, for example, at high temperatures, like boiling or pressure cooking, will inactivate these substances. In addition, soaking them overnight or for several hours should help neutralize them. Studies show that cooked lectin-containing food is safe to consume since exposure to high temperatures has eliminated or reduced the lectin content.

Other methods that will reduce lectin levels are, for example, sprouting and fermenting. Sprouted and fermented beans, grains, and seeds contain less lectin than if unsprouted or unfermented. Removing the outer shell is a good idea when eating nuts since the outside cover has most of the compounds. Some recommend using natural lectin inhibitors when consuming lectin-rich foods.

These natural lectin inhibitors include okra, kiwi, and cranberries. These foods have or stimulate the production of substances that block lectins in the body ("Five Natural ," 2023).

Gluten

Gluten is a protein in grains like wheat, barley, and rye. The problem with these foods is that they can activate an immune reaction in people with celiac disease. Celiac disease is an autoimmune condition that impairs the small intestine's lining and interferes with nutrient absorption.

Gluten sensitivity, contrary to celiac disease, is known as non-celiac gluten sensitivity (NCGS), and this term is used to describe health problems associated with consuming these foods. Symptoms of NCGS are comparable to celiac disease; however, while gluten sensitivity may result in minor intestinal impairment, the damage caused by celiac disease can be extensive. It's recommended to eliminate all gluten products if suffering from this disorder. But just a reduction of gluten will result in an improvement when gluten sensitivity is the problem.

Interestingly, gluten-containing foods are also high in fructans, one of the fermentable oligosaccharides in FODMAPs. Because of this overlap, a gluten-free diet may help improve IBS symptoms.

However, people who tolerate gluten don't need to avoid it; a gluten-free diet tends to be low in fiber and, instead, rich in simple carbohydrates, additives, and fats. It may also result in low levels of other nutrients like folate and vitamin D.

Soy

Soy is a high protein source found in soybeans. It has long been used as a meat substitute for its protein content and other nutrients. The isoflavones in soy have been a traditional remedy for menopause symptoms in some areas of the world, but isoflavones, or phytoestrogen substances, have estrogenic and antiestrogenic effects. So, these compounds can cause physiological effects similar to the hormone estrogen in the body.

In recent years, soy has become more popular as part of alternative healthcare and natural remedies. The consumption of soy or isoflavones can be controversial. Studies agree with its benefits for menopausal symptom management and have also found that it can prevent cardiovascular disease and some cancers (Chen et al., 2021). However, there is a belief that phytoestrogens and soy consumption can cause the possible stimulation of tumor development, increasing the risk of breast cancer. Still, this theory doesn't seem to have been confirmed by any study ("Does Soy Cause Cancer?", 2021).

In addition to being associated with negatively impacting estrogen levels in the body, soy is also rich in lectins and the FODMAP galacto-oligosaccharides. For instance, these substances can sometimes trigger intestinal irritation and cause digestive symptoms typical in IBS conditions.

Despite the negative implications of soy consumption, its multiple benefits, such as being high in protein, fiber, and antioxidants, are undeniable. Moderate soy consumption several times a week is considered safe, assuming our bodies tolerate it. And, in some forms, soy products are low in FODMAP due to their processing: the processing of firm tofu helps in the removal of fermentable sugars; soy milk is made from the soy protein instead of the bean, and tempeh is also low in FODMAP due to the fermentation process.

Nightshades

Nightshades are a family of vegetables containing solanine, an alkaloid, or an organic nitrogen compound. Alkaloids, if consumed in large quantities, are considered dangerous.

Common nightshade foods include white potatoes, eggplants, tomatoes, goji berries, okra, and peppers. These foods contain antioxidants and vitamins and are an excellent fiber source.

Nightshade foods are commonly low in FODMAPs. Although there's no substantial evidence that nightshades cause health issues, some claim these foods can trigger an inflammatory response in our bodies. Sensitive people may experience digestive issues like IBS, IBD, and leaky gut syndrome. Nerve problems such as joint pain, arthritis, allergies, autoimmunity, or other chronic conditions are also associated with nightshade sensitivity ("How nightshades," n.d.).

Dairy

Dairy refers to milk or products made from the milk of cows and goats, for example. Milk products can be high in saturated fats and cholesterol content. They also contain lactose, the disaccharide in the FODMAP classification. The enzyme lactase is required to break down this sugar in our small intestine.

If lactose intolerant, we may not produce enough of this enzyme, resulting in bacteria fermenting lactose in the large intestine. Gas, bloating, and diarrhea will typically follow. Lactose intolerance seems to be common in people suffering from IBS.

Casein, a protein in dairy, might be another allergy source for some. It can trigger allergic reactions such as skin rashes and swelling if sensitive to it.

What about fermented dairy products such as yogurt or kefir? Yogurt is made from warm milk fermented with good bacteria including lactobacillus and bifidobacterium. Kefir is the result of fermenting milk using kefir grains, which are colonies of multiple strains of bacteria and yeast; therefore, kefir contains a more diverse source of probiotics and has higher calcium levels than yogurt. Although yogurt and kefir are considered high in FODMAPs, in some cases, Greek yogurt, in small quantities, is accepted as low in FODMAPs. As for kefir, its process is usually longer than when making yogurt; thus, its lactose content is reduced.

For those who tolerate dairy foods, kefir and yogurt can be an excellent addition to our diet. Choosing plain yogurt and kefir with no additives like sugar, flavors, and colors will benefit our health most.

Histamines

Histamines are organic substances produced naturally in our body and have a role in immune responses that can result in inflammation, allergies, and pain. They're antibodies secreted in response to what our immune system considers invaders, such as bacteria or viruses or other substances or particles like pollen.

Histamines can act as a hormone because they can communicate messages to the brain to activate gastric secretions and expand blood vessels to lower blood pressure, for instance.

It's related to estrogen; higher estrogen levels can trigger histamine production, and histamines can increase estrogen levels (Liu et al., 2018).

Although histamines are primarily produced in our bodies, some foods contain them, too. These include fermented foods and beverages like kombucha, yogurt, alcohol, processed meats, shellfish, legumes, tomatoes, and eggplants.

Histamine intolerance can occur when the body doesn't produce the enzyme needed to break down histamines from food, resulting in digestive issues, headaches, fatigue, or nasal congestion. Avoiding trigger foods or taking enzyme supplements can be advantageous in these situations. In addition, vitamin C and the supplement Quercetin, an antioxidant, can help reduce the production of histamines in the body (Mlcek et al., 2016).

As we saw in this chapter, most typical diets can be adapted to our digestive needs. By knowing the potential impact specific foods can have on our health, we can choose whether to consume or avoid them or modify how we incorporate them into our daily meals. Generally, a well-balanced diet that includes healthy proteins, fats, and plant-based foods that promote our gut micro-biota will positively impact our digestive well-being.

8

THE BENEFITS OF REDUCING STRESS

S tress, we all know how it feels. It's that feeling of being ready to snap or so wound up we can't sleep or eat. It can be the dread of going to work, school, or the daily commute.

But stress isn't always bad; it can be helpful in certain situations. For example, it helps us deal with emergencies and meet deadlines. But when stress becomes chronic, it can cause problems for our bodies. It's an inevitable part of life, and the issue becomes when too much harms our health. Chronic stress can trigger anxiety disorders, depression, heart disease, and gut diseases.

Since the gut and the brain are so closely related, any chronic change in the brain reflects in our digestive health and perhaps more directly than other organs. Fortunately, there are steps we can take to minimize its impact. We need to adopt measures to reduce our stress levels.

PHYSICAL ACTIVITY

Physical activity is an important component of a healthy life-style. It helps us feel better, manage weight, and maintain a healthy heart. And of course, it can also help us reduce stress levels, which is extremely important in managing IBS and other digestive conditions. Low to moderate-intensity activities like brisk walks or yoga can help relieve gastrointestinal symptoms, particularly constipation.

YOGA

Yoga is a spiritual practice that began in India over 5,000 years ago. Yoga combines physical postures, breathing techniques, and meditation to help relax and reduce stress. Yoga can help cope with stress by switching the nervous system into a parasympathetic mode, which allows it to relax and rest. The parasympathetic mode is also part of the nervous system that promotes rest and digestion. When this system is activated, it slows down the heart rate and sends blood flow toward the gut for the proper digestion of food.

Yoga also works by rhythmic, systemic contraction and relaxation of the muscles. This relaxation state helps peristalsis, or food movement in the digestive tract, reducing constipation and fermentation as the food passes through the large intestine. Yoga also helps in increasing blood supply to the gut and reducing inflammation. Studies show that practicing yoga regularly for only six months can reduce IBS symptoms (Kavuri et al., 2015).

One of the key aspects of yoga is breathing. Inhaling and exhaling through the nose should be deep but effortless and relaxed. The inhalation causes the upper body to lift or extend. This action helps deepen the posture during exhalation, as it occurs in bending or twisting positions.

These are some helpful yoga poses:

Downward-Facing Dog:

A downward-facing dog has many benefits. Aside from aiding digestion, it stretches the hamstrings and calf muscles, lengthening the spine, increasing arm strength and shoulder flexibility, and improving balance. It also helps to increase blood circulation all over the body.

To do the Pose:

- Get in plank or tabletop position (hands and feet on the floor if plank or hands and knees if tabletop).
- Tuck toes under and lift the hips while keeping the weight on the feet and palms. Straighten the legs, but keep the knees slightly bent if not possible to straighten. Try to bring your heels to the floor.
- Hold the pose for 20 to 30 seconds.

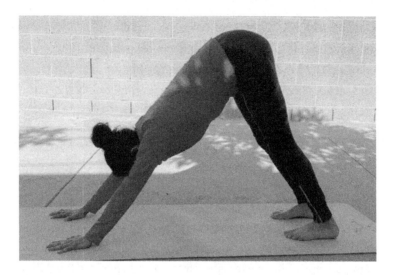

Caution:

While doing the pose, keep the back straight and avoid rounding it.

This pose may not be recommended during pregnancy or for people suffering from back, hamstring, or wrist injuries.

Don't overstretch; bend only as long as the stretching feels comfortable.

Wind Relieving:

This pose strengthens the back, arms, shoulders, thighs, hips, and abdomen, which helps to relieve tension. It massages internal organs and can help with abdominal pain, bloating, and releasing gas.

To do the Pose:

- Start by lying on your back straight on the floor.
- Bend both knees (or one at a time) and pull them up to the chest.
- Wrap the hands around the leg(s) and tightly press the knees and thighs to the chest.
- Hold the pose for 20-60 seconds or three to five breaths and release the legs to the ground.
- Repeat with the other leg if doing one at a time.

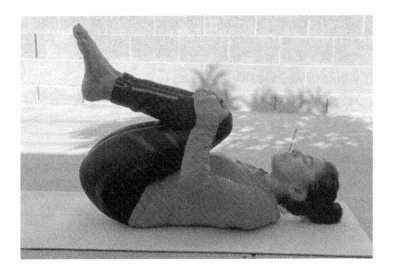

Caution:

Avoid this pose if recovering from abdominal surgery, have back injuries, or during pregnancy.

Half-Seated Spinal Twist:

The half-seated spinal twist is a gentle and relaxing stretch. It has beneficial effects on the digestive organs. It stimulates the large intestine and aids in constipation.

To do the Pose:

- Sit up straight on the floor with legs extended in front.
- Bend the left leg, bring it over to the outside of the right leg, and plant the foot next to the left thigh/knee.
- Bend the right knee and bring the leg back until the right ankle is next to the left gluteus (you could also keep the left leg straight in front).
- Put the left hand behind your back on the floor.
- Raise the right arm and lower the hand or elbow to rest on the bent left knee while twisting the upper body and facing the left.
- Inhale, and try to twist further to the left with each exhalation.
- Hold 5-10 breaths and then repeat on the other side.

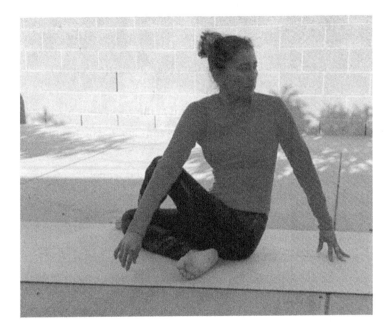

Caution:

Caution should be observed during menstruation or pregnancy.
Avoid if suffering a hernia, peptic ulcers, or back/spinal injuries.

Seated Forward Bend:

The seated forward bend is a classic yoga pose that stretches the
hamstrings and the lower back. It helps relieve stress and anxiety
and aids digestion by stimulating the liver and kidneys.

To do the Pose:

- Start by sitting up straight with both legs extended in front.
- Then, as exhaling, bend forward at the waist and slowly lower the torso, hinging from the hips and trying to grab feet or toes.
- Only bend as far as it is comfortable and without rounding the back.
- If very flexible, bend until the face presses against the knees and thighs.
- Hold this pose for 30 seconds to one minute while inhaling and exhaling normally; try to bend further with each exhale.

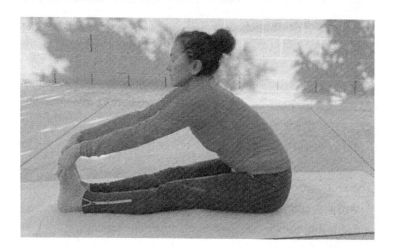

Caution:

Avoid this pose during pregnancy and if suffering hip, hamstring, or back injuries.

Cat and Cow:

Cat and cow pose are two of the most popular poses in yoga, and they're great for digestive health and help to improve the flexibility of the back and relieve stress. They also massage internal organs like the kidney and adrenal glands and aid digestion by easing bloating and abdominal pain.

To do the Pose:

- Start on all fours with hands and knees on the floor: knees below the hips and wrists below the shoulders; the spine is neutral.
- For the cow pose: in the inhalation, lift the head and gaze, and arch the back downwards toward the ground.
- For the cat pose: in the exhalation, curl the back, rounding the spine upward and chin toward the chest.
- Continue alternating between both poses and complete about ten repetitions.

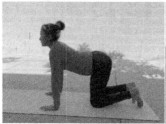 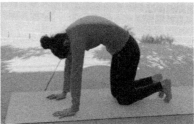

Caution:

This pose may not be recommended or should be performed cautiously if suffering knee, neck, or back problems.

Child's Pose:

The child's pose is excellent for relieving tension in the lower back, lengthening the spine, and improving blood circulation. It also stimulates the organs and promotes digestion, as it can alleviate pain and release gas.

To do the Pose:

- Start kneeling; feet are close together, and big toes are touching. The knees can be wide open.
- Sit back onto the heels and lower the upper body to rest between or over the thighs.
- Rest the forehead on the floor in front and extend the arms forward.
- Hold the pose for 20-60 seconds.

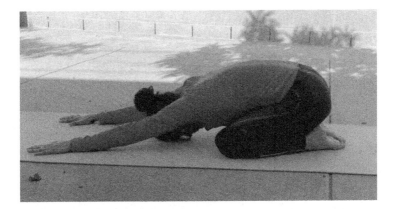

Caution:

- Avoid this pose if suffer from diarrhea, high blood pressure, or injury to the spine, neck, feet, thighs, and knees.

Cobra:

This pose is excellent for stretching the lower back, increasing blood supply to the intestines, and aiding in constipation.

- Lie on your stomach with your forehead on the ground, your legs extended behind, and the top of your feet touching the mat.
- Press the palms against the floor by the shoulders, fingertips facing the front of the mat.
- Lift the head and chest while bending the elbows to the side, close to the body.

- Head and chest should be off the floor with palms pressing on the mat.
- Slowly straighten the elbows, lift the upper body off the floor, and keep the palms, pelvic area, thighs, and feet touching the mat.
- Hold the pose for 30 seconds, then lower the body to the ground on the exhalation.
- Repeat about five more time.

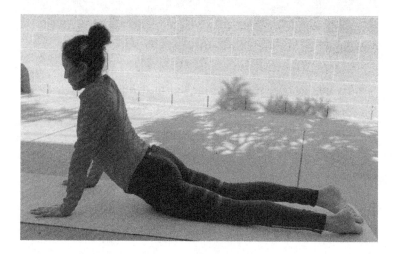

Caution:

This pose isn't recommended during pregnancy. Also, avoid it if you have any wrists, shoulders, back, or arms injuries or are recovering from abdominal surgery.

Bow:

Bow pose is excellent for stretching the abdominal muscles, putting pressure on the abdomen, increasing blood flow, and aiding in gastrointestinal disorders. It also helps in easing menstrual pain.

To do the Pose:

- Lie down on the stomach, arms at the sides, palms facing up toward the back of the mat.
- Bend the knees, prop the feet in the air, and grab the ankles.
- Lift the head and shoulders gently off the floor while keeping the lower back flat and resting on the belly.
- Lift the thighs while holding the ankles with the hands.
- Hold for 10 to 15 seconds while breathing normally.

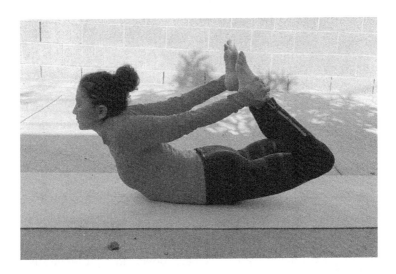

Caution:

This pose isn't recommended during pregnancy or menstruation. It's also not recommended if you suffer from high blood pressure, have an injury to the neck or back, or had abdominal surgery recently.

WALKING

Like yoga, walking is an excellent way to relieve anxiety and stress. It's easy to do, can be done anywhere, doesn't require special equipment or training, and can be done any time of the day or night.

If we suffer from IBS, regular walking sessions may help relieve symptoms (Shahabi et al., 2015). This effect is partly due to its ability to help regulate bowel movements. It also helps ease digestion by increasing blood flow and oxygen levels in the colon, which improves digestion.

MEDITATION

Meditation is a practice that can aid in reducing stress and improving overall health. It's a tool that helps manage emotions, thoughts, and behaviors. Meditation can also be a way to connect more profoundly with oneself and others.

The brain and gut have a strong connection, and when the brain is relaxed, it stops the constant state of survival mode (fight or flight response of the nervous system). In a relaxed state, our brain isn't sending stress signals down the gut-brain axis anymore. The temporary halting of stress signals is why meditation can help with symptoms of digestive issues.

Meditation also helps in maintaining gut microbiome health as gut bacteria play a huge part in making neurotransmitters related to mood, like serotonin. So, an imbalanced gut microbiome hinders our emotional state.

The opposite is true, however: our moods affect the gut microbiome. Research shows meditation can help reduce gut disorders like IBS and IBD by regulating our emotions. During this Harvard research, they found that reflection (or relaxation response) was helpful to the participants in two ways: first, it reduced the expression of several genes directly linked to the main inflammatory processes of IBD, and second, it helped them control their response to stressful conditions and become more resilient to pain and stress (Kuo et al., 2015).

There are many types of meditation, but they all have one objective: to find inner peace or relaxation ("Mayo Clinic," 2020).

Guided: In this type of meditation, we practice visualization, where we mentally form images of places or situations that relax us, like walking in a beautiful garden or forest, smelling flowers, or listening to bird sounds. Often, in this type of meditation, an instructor guides us. If not, we could play audio that describes what we're seeing, hearing, smelling, or touching.

Mindful: Mindful meditation requires us to be aware of the present moment. During this meditation, we can focus on how we feel at each moment: our breath or emotions, for example.

But the key is to let this go without judging what we're experiencing at that moment.

Transcendental: This is a technique where, in silence, we repeat a mantra in a certain way, like chanting. This mantra can be a word or a phrase that can distract us from constant thinking. A common Hindu mantra is "Om," which is thought to be the sound of the universe. There are other Hindu mantras, but we can choose positive phrases instead.

Meditation has some essential elements. First, we need to be comfortable, usually seated, but it can be done lying down or walking. Focus is an important feature as this will help us free our mind from the distractions and thoughts that are often causing us stress. Our breathing should be deep and relaxed. Often, just focusing on our breathing can be our meditation. The place where we meditate should be quiet; when we're beginners, this is important since we aren't used to tuning out distractions yet.

COGNITIVE BEHAVIORAL TECHNIQUE (CBT)

The cognitive behavioral technique (CBT) is a short-term, skill-based therapy that focuses on modifying behavior and altering dysfunctional thinking patterns to influence mood and physiological symptoms.

CBT is often used as a first-line therapy for IBS because it's easy to learn, effective for many patients, and the therapist can tailor it for individual needs. One benefit of CBT is that it improves the quality of life by reducing psychological distress and improving coping skills for patients with IBS ("Cognitive Behavioral," 2021).

Healthy, thought-out cognitive behavioral therapy includes a psychoeducational component, which provides patients with information about the biology of IBS, the brain-gut axis, physiological stress response, and the basis for the behavioral approach. This method focuses on relaxation strategies that help patients activate their parasympathetic nervous system. Patients also learn about physical tensions, stressors, and anxiety management. A cognitive restructuring component is the key to helping the patient recognize distorted thinking patterns and their relationship with stress and digestive symptoms. Problem-solving techniques are the part that teaches the patients how to cope with stressful situations. Finally, exposure techniques are used in therapy to help patients face problems they usually avoid because they may trigger the symptoms.

HYPNOSIS

Hypnosis helps us focus on our symptoms and calm the digestive tract to prevent unnecessary discomfort. It's more of a guided relaxation for people who find it difficult to let go independently. In hypnosis, a therapist guides patients into a focused state of awareness while keeping them relaxed. This process helps them to address the miscommunication between the gut and the brain. Research indicates hypnosis may help improve the symptoms of IBS ("Hypnosis for IBS," n. d.).

In conclusion, stress-relieving techniques will tremendously impact our digestive condition. A simple walk or some yoga will help improve peristaltic contractions and reduce inflammation. Meditation, hypnosis, and cognitive behavioral techniques are possible alternatives for relieving IBS and other digestive disorders.

9

NUTRITIONAL SUPPLEMENTS, HERBAL REMEDIES, AND ALTERNATIVE APPROACHES

The human body is a complex machine. And while we're all aware of the importance of consuming good foods, one area we may need to pay attention to is the amount of nutrients we consume and how often.

That isn't to say we have to take supplements to lead a healthy lifestyle. But when we notice that our body, especially the gut, and hormones, have been feeling a little off, it might be time to add some supplements into our daily routine. Supplements and herbal remedies have an overall and far-reaching effect over medications.

However, the wide selection of supplements claiming to be the cure-all can be intimidating, and it often takes time to understand where to start.

The following is a list of commonly recommended products to improve digestive health.

PREBIOTICS

Prebiotics are non-digestible carbohydrates that promote the activity of bacteria or feed these microorganisms in our gut. This fiber-like sugar compound doesn't get broken down or absorbed in the intestines; instead, it ferments, producing butyric acid critical for healthy digestive cells. The acid production helps maintain a balanced pH in the colon, and the acidic conditions are ideal for beneficial bacteria and keeping pathogens away. Prebiotics also increase bifidobacterium. This helpful microorganism is useful in reducing inflammation and helps in the digestion of fiber. IBS sufferers generally have a low amount of this bacteria ("Best Probiotics," 2017).

Prebiotics are fiber; however, not all fiber is prebiotic. Several plant-based foods, including everyday herbs like ginger, onion, leeks, asparagus, and grains like barley and oats, are rich in prebiotics. In addition to providing the benefits of fiber, these foods offer many other nutrients like almonds, which can help to improve memory, and pomegranates, which have many antioxidants and vitamin C.

Unfortunately, prebiotics are found primarily in foods high in FODMAP, like fructans and Galacto-Oligosaccharides, common in garlic, onion, legumes, and grains. But the good news is that these high-FODMAP prebiotic foods are often tolerable in small quantities, and these quantities are adaptable according to symptoms.

There are also prebiotic foods that are low in FODMAPs. These include fennel, eggplants, grapefruit, pomegranate, kiwi, almonds, and oats.

Prebiotics can also be taken as supplements, starting with a low dose if fiber consumption in the regular diet has been minimal.

- About 5 grams per day is considered a safe dose
- The best time to take it is often in the morning, at bedtime, or on an empty stomach,
- It can be taken together with probiotics.

Although prebiotics can improve digestive health, in some people, especially if taken in large amounts, they can cause bloating and gas (Marteau et al., 2004).

PROBIOTICS

Probiotics are specific strains of beneficial bacteria. These microorganisms are alive and add to the good bacterial colonies that already exist in our bodies. Probiotics have become increasingly popular as research proves their potential health benefits. Among its benefits is that they can help calm symptoms of abdominal pain, especially if these are due to bacterial imbalance, as these bacteria are helpful in restoring the microbiota balance. Thus, they can help treat IBS and the symptoms of IBD (Didari et al., 2015).

Probiotics are found in food and also as supplements. Lactobacillus and bifidobacterial are the most common strains. If a product names only one type, it's usually Lactobacillus acidophilus, which is generally the most effective for health purposes. Saccharomyces boulardii is another strain considered helpful in reducing diarrhea symptoms.

Yogurt and kefir are popular probiotic foods. But there are non-dairy options available, like coconut yogurt. Greek yogurt is often deemed more tolerable because much of its lactose content has been removed during the additional processing. The same can be said for kefir. Kefir contains more probiotic strains than yogurt.

- Probiotic supplements are usually available in 1 to 10 billion cell counts. Doses of 50 billion or higher are also available.
- When starting to consume probiotics, a low dose is often recommended; then, we should assess how our body reacts and adjust the dose accordingly.
- The best time to take it is usually at bedtime or before meals on an empty stomach, about 30 minutes before eating.
- Probiotics and prebiotics can be taken together.

Probiotics can provide excellent benefits for digestion in some people. However, in others, they can have the opposite effect; bloating, diarrhea, and unrelated symptoms like dizziness and headaches can be experienced.

FERMENTED FOODS

Fermentation is an ancient technique of food preservation in which microorganisms eat sugars and produce acids and alcohol. That's why it's often associated with wine and beer.

The strains of bacteria needed for fermentation are variable, but the ones in the food may not be active once they enter the digestive tract. Although it's a less reliable method of promoting our friendly bacteria, fermented foods have many benefits: aside from fermentation stopping food from spoiling quickly (which makes it such a good preservation technique), it also makes food easier to digest because the bacteria break down sugars into smaller molecules so foods like kombucha, kimchi, and sauerkraut, are still a good source of good bacteria (Nielsen et al., 2018).

Like probiotics, some people may not tolerate fermented foods well and can experience common digestive symptoms, headaches, and histamine intolerance. Histamines are chemical compounds that trigger allergies. Our bodies produce them, but fermented foods can also be high in these substances.

DIGESTIVE ENZYMES

Digestive enzymes are proteins made mainly in the pancreas and intestines. They're needed to break down food into smaller particles for better absorption into our bodies. Common digestive enzymes are amylase, lipase, lactase, and protease; these break down carbohydrates, fats, lactose, and proteins.

Supplementation of digestive enzymes is sometimes necessary if enzymatic production in our body is insufficient. For example, lactose intolerance may occur when undigested lactose particles pass to the colon, where they get fermented, causing diarrhea and other symptoms. In this case, supplementing with lactase or adhering to a diet that includes tolerable dairy FODMAP products is recommended.

Alpha-galactosidase is another enzyme that can potentially improve the absorption of galactan oligosaccharide substances, typically found in legumes.

Other enzymes, like bromelain and papain, are naturally found in pineapple and papaya. These are known as proteolytic enzymes and can help break down proteins. These have a role in reducing inflammation, pain, and swelling and can also help in improving digestive symptoms. Fermented foods, kiwi, ginger, and asparagus, also contain proteolytic enzymes.

- Enzymes are also available in tablets, powder, or capsules.
- These are often taken at the beginning of a meal.
- Like many other supplements, they may cause side effects like allergies and digestive discomfort.

BONE BROTH

Bone broth is a nutritious food that usually has the consistency of gelatin. It's made by boiling animal bones, usually from chicken or beef, and connective tissues that contain many vitamins and minerals. In addition to tasting great, bone broth has numerous health benefits. It's high in collagen and amino acids, excellent for treating leaky gut and ulcers and calming IBS symptoms. Also, collagen is known for its anti-inflammatory properties and promoting good bacteria.

Beef bone broth, as opposed to chicken bone broth, is considered higher in nutritional value because it contains more minerals and the amino acid glycine. Glycine is crucial for our gut and helps form collagen type III, a significant component for internal organs; this helps support digestive health.

One of the ways to prepare bone broth is to roast bones for about 2-3 hours. This process enhances its flavor and texture. The roasted bones can then be cooked in a large pot with water and herbs and simmered for 5-8 hours or longer. One to two cups per day can be consumed daily.

Although considered highly advantageous for our health, bone broth has a high glutamate content, which can cause sensitivities in some due to the glutamate properties to enhance histamine release. Some people may experience headaches, allergies, anxiety, indigestion, and joint pain.

GLUTAMINE

Glutamine (not the same as glutamate) is a naturally occurring amino acid that supports intestinal health. Most of the body's glutamine is in muscle tissue, but it also makes up a high percentage of the free amino acids in the small intestine.

Since glutamine plays a vital role in intestinal inflammatory signaling pathways, protecting cells against apoptosis (programmed cell death), inducing cell proliferation, and preventing cellular stress, it's considered one of the essential nutrients for maintaining proper gut function. Supplementation with this amino acid may benefit IBD sufferers. Glutamine may also help decrease symptoms of IBS.

High-protein foods like meats, seafood, and eggs are rich in glutamine. Leafy greens can also promote glutamine production in our bodies.

- Glutamine in a supplement form is commonly available as L-Glutamine in capsules, tablets, or powder.
- The powder form is often a better option due to its higher absorption rate.
- Doses of 5 grams daily are considered safe.
- It should be taken on an empty stomach before meals for best results.

Similar to other supplements, some people may experience side effects when consuming glutamine. These symptoms may include dizziness, nausea, skin rashes or itchiness, inflammation of hands and feet, and joint pain.

GLUTATHIONE

Glutathione, made of amino acids mainly in our liver, is a critical compound for many reasons. It acts as an antioxidant, neutralizing the damage caused by oxidative stress (a condition in our body when there are too many free radicals and not enough antioxidants). It's also vital to ensure that our immune system works correctly, particularly for T cells. This white cell helps protect the body from infections.

In addition to environmental factors such as diet and stress, our glutathione levels drop as we age. As a result, older adults more frequently develop inflammation-related diseases, like allergies and arthritis, or cancer cells that grow out of control more easily. Although glutathione isn't a cure-all (nothing is), it's a powerful antioxidant and works excellently against leaky gut and other inflammatory conditions like IBD.

Consuming sulfur-rich foods like cruciferous vegetables, including broccoli or kale, will increase glutathione levels in our bodies.

Foods rich in vitamin C, protein, and exercise can also help with glutathione production.

- Glutathione is often available as a supplement in powder, liquid, capsules, and even in intravenous or intramuscular forms.
- One gram is considered a safe dose.
- The best time to take it would be on an empty stomach before meals.

Studies, however, indicate that if consumed orally, glutathione is absorbed poorly in our body (Sharma et al., 2022).

Some people experience side effects like abdominal cramps, allergies, and bloating.

OILS

Coconut oil/MCT

We are likely aware of the health benefits of coconut oil, but sometimes we may not understand why certain fats are healthy, and others aren't. The significant difference is the length of the fatty acid chain—the chain that makes up the building blocks of triglycerides, a type of fat. Its high content of medium-chain triglycerides (MCTs), which are metabolized differently and faster than long-chain triglycerides, is what makes MCTs rich in health benefits.

Among the health benefits is that it increases short-chain fatty acids (like butyrate) in our intestines, reduces harmful bacteria and inflammation, and improves microbiota and intestinal functioning.

It's also high in lauric acid, converted into monolaurin in the body. Monolaurin is known to fight dangerous viruses such as HIV and herpes. These excellent properties make coconut oil a potent tool for fighting harmful pathogens in the gut (Jia et al., 2020).

Virgin and cold-pressed forms are often recommended for maximum benefits, but 100% MCT oil is more potent than regular oil. Due to its quick conversion to ketone bodies, produced by the liver when glucose is unavailable, MCT oil consumption during keto diets could provide better results.

Coconut oil is also a healthy choice for cooking due to its high smoking point ("SCL Health," 2018), and it can be added to warm beverages, smoothies, or shakes.

One of the drawbacks is that up to 90% of coconut oil fat content is considered saturated, and this type of fat tends to increase cholesterol and triglycerides. But one tablespoon per day is considered safe and low in FODMAP.

Olive oil

Olive oil is also a healthy fat with many uses. It can be great for smoothies, salad dressings, or drizzled-over food. It's rich in polyphenol antioxidants. It decreases inflammation, and some of its components are prebiotics, which feed the good digestive bacteria in the gut and helps produce short-chain fatty acids that provide nutrients to the cells lining the intestines. It may also reduce symptoms of colitis. This oil has natural laxative properties; therefore, it stimulates bowel movements.

Cold-pressed and the extra virgin form are considered healthier options, and taking one to two tablespoons per day can provide benefits. Taking one tablespoon on an empty stomach in the morning for constipation may help alleviate this condition.

The use of olive oil in cooking is debatable; some contend that heat damages its beneficial compounds because, compared to other oils, it has a lower smoking point, which is the point where the oil starts to break down. The smoking point of olive oil, based on the type (refined, virgin, extra virgin), can vary between 320 and 470 degrees.

Others consider olive oil one of the most stable due to its monosaturated fat content, which makes it safe to expose to heat ("About Olive Oil," 2018).

But like any other fat, excessive consumption can result in extra calories since fats have a higher calorie content than carbohydrates or proteins.

Oregano oil

Oregano oil is an excellent source of antioxidants, which fight free radicals in the body. Free radicals can damage older cells, which causes inflammation and swelling. This oil contains thymol, an active ingredient used to treat fungal infections and parasites. It's also effective in treating some types of bacteria that cause digestive issues, like SIBO and H. pylori (Helicobacter pylori), which are associated with ulcers, gastritis, and stomach cancer. It's a natural alternative to antibiotics.

Like other essential oils, oregano oil is only as good as its quality—so buying a 100% therapeutic-grade form is a safer option.

- It shouldn't be used alone, topical, or ingested, as it can burn the skin. Instead, it should be diluted with water or olive or coconut oil.
- The recommended dosage is between two and four daily drops, depending on the brand.
- It may also be available in capsule forms.

Also, using for extended periods (more than a week) or in large doses should be avoided, or take breaks in between uses to prevent toxicity. It should be avoided during pregnancy or if preparing for surgery. Higher doses may cause allergies, stomach issues, headaches, and dizziness ("LiverTox," 2023).

Black seed oil

Black seed oil is from the seeds of the plant Nigella Sativa, and it has been part of traditional medicine since ancient times. It has a potent active compound named Thymoquinone. It's an antioxidant and has anti-allergy, anti-inflammatory, and immune-supporting properties.

One of the uses of black seed oil is to support digestion: it decreases bloating, gas, and stomach pain, so it can help if you suffer from IBS or IBD as it suppresses inflammation.

- Opt for cold-pressed, pure, therapeutic grade, and organic formulas when choosing black seed oil.
- It's often available in capsules, oil, and seeds or powder.
- One gram is considered a safe dose. However, up to 2

grams daily is advisable for up to three months
("BLACK SEED," n.d.).

Avoiding black seed oil during pregnancy is recommended. It could trigger allergic reactions, be toxic in large doses, and slow blood clotting.

Omega-3

Omega-3 is an essential fatty acid that aids our body fight inflammatory diseases. It helps to lower the risk of heart problems, promotes a healthy and diverse microbiome, and discourages the growth of harmful bacteria, ultimately keeping inflammation at bay (Costantini et al., 2017).

The amount of omega-3 in our body depends on our diet. Our bodies can't produce it, so we need to get it from food sources. One of the best sources is fish, but it's also present in plant-based foods like flax and chia seeds and their oils.

- A recommended dose is up to 2 grams per day.

Some people experience acid reflux or other digestive symptoms and may experience blood thinning.

OTHER ESSENTIAL SUPPLEMENTS:

Vitamin D

Vitamin D, a fat-soluble vitamin, helps control calcium and phosphorus levels in our blood by increasing intestinal absorption from food and supplements like magnesium and zinc. It also has anti-inflammatory properties and acts on the GI tract through various mechanisms. It helps protect against certain gastrointestinal diseases, including IBD, celiac disease, and colon cancer. It also has anti-inflammatory and immune-modulating effects on the digestive tract and regulates the gut microbiome (Akimbekov et al., 2020).

We find vitamin D in salmon, tuna, eggs, and red meat. Non-food sources are exposure to sun and supplementation. For people suffering from IBS, supplementing vitamin D is necessary since deficiency tends to be prevalent if suffering from this condition.

- As a supplement, its popular form is D3, and recommended doses are around 2000 IU daily.

Vitamin D can be fatal if consumed in excess. Doses of 40,000–100,000 IU daily are considered unsafe for extended periods. However, high doses are acceptable for short periods if levels in the body are low. Excess vitamin D may result in kidney stones, dehydration, nausea, or irritability.

Vitamin C

Vitamin C, or Ascorbic acid, is a necessary nutrient for humans. It helps maintain a balance between good and bad bacteria and increases diversity in the gut. Vitamin C plays a significant role in anti-inflammatory processes in the body, so it's no surprise that some people with chronic inflammation have found relief by supplementing vitamin C. It can help improve gut barrier functions and increase stomach acid production. It's also essential for healthy bones and teeth, helps produce collagen that keeps our skin and connective tissues strong, heals wounds, increases energy levels, and improves mood. Osteoporosis is a common condition in people with IBS; the low consumption of vegetables and fruits, high in vitamin C, often eliminated during a low FODMAP diet, is probably one cause (Ratajczak et al., 2020).

Ascorbic acid is found in citrus fruits, potatoes, tomatoes, bell peppers, and cruciferous vegetables.

- In supplement forms, it's available in tablets, powder, intravenous, liquid, and capsules.
- Time-release formulas are released slowly throughout, so it has better bioavailability.
- Some formulas are buffered with added alkalinizing effects to reduce their acidity. Buffered formulas are considered more soothing on the stomach and have increased absorption.
- Vitamin C is safe to take on an empty stomach before food.

- Recommended doses are up to 2 grams daily, and higher quantities are safe for short periods.

Taking excessively or for extended periods may have laxative effects and cause nausea, diarrhea, and stomach aches.

HERBAL REMEDIES

Licorice root

Licorice root, or "the sweet herb," is native to Europe and Asia. It has a long history of medicinal use to treat many ailments, including the common cold and stomach ulcers. In Ayurvedic medicine, licorice root helps to alleviate heartburn and ulcers while reducing inflammation.

The active ingredient in licorice root is glycyrrhizin. This substance works by helping the body produce natural anti-inflammatory and immune system regulators. Licorice root helps decrease H. pylori counts in the stomach, indicating that it could help treat H. pylori-induced gastritis and peptic ulcers. It may also help reduce heartburn and GERD symptoms and benefit asthma and other respiratory infections (Authier et al., 2022). It's helpful in hormone health as it can ease menstruation and menopausal symptoms.

- It is available as cut/woody pieces, powder, extract, capsules, and teas

- It can be used by itself or combined with other herbs to make beverages or tinctures.
- Under 1 gram is considered a safe dose.

Overusing licorice may lead to edema, high blood pressure, low potassium levels, and chronic fatigue. It can cause estrogen-like effects on female hormones, leading to hormonal imbalances.

Slippery elm

This herb comes from the bark of the slippery elm tree, which grows all over North America. The inner part of the bark has lots of mucilage similar to the inside of the stomach and digestive tract. When ingested, it coats the gastrointestinal lining with a slippery coating ("Slippery Elm," n. d.).

It also stimulates the GI tract's reflux, increasing mucous secretion. This substance acts as a preventive barrier and protects the mucosa against ulcers and excess acidity. When the stomach acidity is somewhat neutralized, it also helps in GERD. Due to its slippery nature, it acts as a laxative and helps with IBD and IBS-C. The antioxidant components of slippery elm help inflammatory bowel conditions. Some believe it helps with vaginal dryness due to its mucous content. The bark's inner layer can be dried up, powdered, and used for constipation.

- Slippery elm comes in capsules, powder, teas, extracts, and tinctures.
- Follow the instructions on the package for the recommended dose.

- Best to take after meals to help with GERD symptoms
  and after meals for lower digestive tract symptoms

Because slippery elm contains a mucus-like substance, it can slow the absorption of other drugs or herbs taken simultaneously. It's not recommended during pregnancy.

Aloe vera

Aloe vera is a plant that we often grow at home. While it's commonly known for its burns and cuts properties, it also does wonders for digestion. The soothing gel from the aloe leaf has laxative properties, making it an effective remedy for constipation. It also contains mucous-like compounds that help protect the gastric mucosa. Its anti-inflammatory properties give it the ability to decrease inflammation ("Aloe Information," n. d.). It also soothes gastric and peptic ulcers and GERD.

When we harvest it directly from the plant, we should use the clear gel rather than the yellowish substance since this can have toxic effects.

- A safe dose is two to three tablespoons of clear gel.
- Aloe is also available in juice or capsules; in these
  forms, it should be consumed only for short periods.

In excess, it can cause diarrhea, allergic reactions, and low blood sugar levels. Aloe may also interfere with the absorption of other medications taken simultaneously.

Mastic gum

Mastic gum, commonly used for sore throats, also benefits gut health. Mastic gum comes from the resin from the pistacia lentiscus tree. The Romans used it as chewing gum for its remedial properties. It has antibacterial, antiviral, and anti-inflammatory qualities and inhibits Helicobacter pylori effects. It prevents ulcers, removes bacteria, and alleviates stomach discomfort (Soulaidopoulos et al., 2020).

It may relieve heartburn and acid reflux by protecting the stomach lining against acid erosions and allowing food to pass quickly. It also alleviates any inflammation caused by GERD.

- Mastic gum is available in capsules, powder, essential oils, and even chewing gum.
- Under 3 grams should be a safe dose for up to three months.

Our body generally tolerates it well, but it can cause headaches, dizziness, and indigestion.

Fennel

Fennel has antioxidant, anti-inflammatory, and antibacterial properties that can help relieve IBS symptoms. Fennel contains essential and volatile (that evaporates quickly) oils. These oils stimulate the secretion of digestive fluids and enzymes. In addition, it could help to relax spasms. The seeds are rich in fiber, which improves digestion. It contains compounds that can aid with hormonal imbalances and help improve menopause symptoms ("WebMD Editorial," 2020).

Fennel bulbs, seeds, and leaves can be eaten raw or cooked. One daily teaspoon of the seeds is safe for consumption.

- As a supplement, it's available in capsules and as an essential oil.

Excess can cause stomach pain, allergic reactions, and vomiting. It may also mimic estrogen, impacting hormone-sensitive conditions like fibroids and breast cancers. It may also slow down blood clotting, increasing the risk of bleeding.

Ginger

Ginger is one of the most common herbal remedies to help improve IBS symptoms. The medicinal use of ginger goes back thousands of years and has a long history of use in Ayurveda and traditional Chinese medicine.

Ginger is a rhizome commonly used to soothe the stomach and help with nausea, vomiting, indigestion, and heartburn. The gingerol ingredient in the herb benefits GI motility and reduces fermentation, constipation, and bloating. It also has anti-inflammatory and antioxidant effects. Specifically, ginger can help with ulcerative colitis and other symptoms like acid reflux, heartburn, nausea, and vomiting associated with pregnancy or other causes (Guo et al., 2021). It has a role in weight loss and aiding the balance of estrogen and other hormones.

The fresh root, or in powder form, is used in food and beverages.

- It's also available in capsules and essential oils.
- A tablespoon of ground ginger or up to 4 grams is considered safe.

In large amounts, it can cause bleeding and low blood sugar. Also, avoiding ginger supplements while taking blood-thinning medications is suggested because the combination might cause bruising.

Turmeric

Turmeric is a perennial herb and a member of the ginger family. It has been part of Indian cooking and Ayurvedic medicine for thousands of years. The herb's root contains curcumin, which is responsible for most turmeric's health benefits.

Curcumin has anti-inflammatory, antioxidant, and antibacterial properties. It relaxes the smooth muscles of the intestines and helps prevent gas and bloating. It also encourages the repairing of a leaky gut.

Curcumin promotes the secretion of stomach mucus, which can help protect against ulcers and help reduce indigestion by encouraging bile production by the liver and gallbladder. As an antioxidant and anti-inflammatory agent, curcumin helps reduce swelling and fights free radicals that contribute to cell damage. Curcumin may also help to prevent cancer by inhibiting tumor growth and helping to regulate genes that suppress tumors (Jurenka, 2009). Studies show curcumin can reduce androgen or male hormones in polycystic ovarian conditions or PCOS.

Turmeric is commonly available as a fresh root or in powder forms. It's typically added to food or beverages like teas, smoothies, or other drinks. Turmeric paste is a homemade or store-bought recipe containing other ingredients. This paste is made by heating or blending raw ingredients. It often includes coconut or olive oil and black pepper to increase curcumin absorption. Other elements like ginger, lemon, and cinnamon are great additions to this paste to improve its nutritional value. One daily teaspoon of this paste can be added to beverages or mixed with food.

- Curcumin is also available in capsules.
- Safe doses are up to 2 grams daily.

Curcumin can slow down blood clotting and cause iron deficiency, low blood sugar, kidney stones, and nausea or diarrhea if consumed in excess.

DAILY HABITS

As we know, many factors contribute to our gut health. It's more than the type of food we eat and the drinks we drink but also how much sleep we get, how active we are, and other daily habits that may tremendously impact our health.

Getting enough sleep

Getting enough sleep is extremely important; less than seven or more than nine hours can lead to irregular bowel movements and stomach pain. Research indicates a strong link between digestive disorders and poor sleep (Khanijow et al., 2015).

Because sleeping is necessary, an established sleep schedule matching our circadian rhythm is essential to maintain a healthy gut. The circadian rhythm is our internal process that controls sleeping and waking cycles, influenced by daylight and darkness.

Being exposed to natural light signals our body that it's time to be awake; darkness helps us relax and activates the production of melatonin, the hormone that induces sleep.

To improve the quality of our sleep, within six hours of bedtime, avoid foods and beverages like caffeine or alcohol. Other typical recommendations include turning off electronic devices, creating a comfortable atmosphere where room temperature, light, and noise are appropriate, practicing relaxation techniques, and avoiding exercising too close to bedtime.

Avoiding processed food

Processed food contains ingredients high in concentration that are harmful to our digestive system; these include added sugars, artificial sweeteners, preservatives, and artificial colors and flavors. These ingredients may adversely affect the microbiome's composition, increasing the risk for IBS and IBD.

Food additives like emulsifiers (carboxymethylcellulose), colors (tartrazine), and preservatives (sulfites) may cause hypersensitive reactions in some IBS patients. Not to mention, a high processed food intake is related to cardiac diseases, diabetes, gut ulcers, and infections.

Chewing food well

In our fast-paced lifestyles, we often don't think chewing food properly is necessary for optimal digestion and overall health. Breaking food into smaller particles through chewing to make a paste will help improve food absorption and digestion.

Chewing stimulates saliva production; saliva contains several digestive agents, including amylase, an enzyme that helps digest carbohydrates, and mucin that coats the mouth and tongue to prevent damage and allow food to go down easily. Chewing also stimulates the production of hydrochloric acid in the stomach. The pH balance is regulated to further assist with the breakdown of food.

Swallowing unchewed food potentially causes heartburn, acid reflux, or other digestive problems. It can also cause bacterial overgrowth, especially when food can't mix with salivary immunoglobulins, antibodies that neutralize toxins and remove harmful microorganisms or pathogens. Chewing food an average of 30 times before swallowing is often recommended.

Eating small meals

Our stomach is a muscular sac with a capacity of around 1-2.5 ounces, depending on its fullness. For the proper digestion and absorption of food, the stomach needs to be able to empty its contents at a specific rate. When we eat large meals or overeat periodically, the stomach frequently stretches beyond its natural size, which can lead to acid reflux.

For optimal digestion, five to six small frequent meals are often recommended as this will help improve digestion, absorb nutrients, and stabilize symptoms of IBS ("IBS Diet," 2021).

In addition, eating smaller portions has the added benefit of fewer calories consumed throughout the day. It also helps balance blood sugar levels and maintain an active metabolism.

Limiting alcohol

Alcohol is known to have devastating effects on the body and brain—like liver disease, an increased risk of cancer, and even depression. But what about that one drink we need to loosen up? Or that one glass of wine to help us unwind after a hard day?

Moderate drinking has some health benefits. But, consuming more than two drinks per day could lead to nasty side effects like acid reflux, bloating, gastritis, damage to the liver and pancreas, reduction of digestive enzyme production, and inflammation and permeability of the intestines. When we drink, bacteria metabolize the alcohol consumed. This process releases toxic byproducts that can inflame the gut and deprive good bacteria of essential nutrients. In addition, it can also lead to bacterial overgrowth and dysbiosis, irritating the intestinal lining, which is associated with flare-ups of IBS and IBD.

———

As we've seen, incorporating other remedies and techniques into our daily regimen is often a significant complement to a healthy lifestyle, where dietary choices and relaxation practices are frequently the primary approaches to finding relief for digestive symptoms. The use of supplements and herbal remedies, as well as making changes to our daily habits and lifestyle, are techniques we should also consider on our path to finding relief.

AUTHOR'S LAST WORD

We have reached the end of the book; a book that I published for you and me. I thank you for getting this far and reading each page (or most of it 😊). Getting this book ready has been a great experience.

I started suffering from digestive issues around thirty, and the doctor diagnosed my condition as IBS. Of course, I followed the traditional advice to treat bloating, constipation, and flatulence. But despite adopting a "healthy" diet and including the often-recommended remedies, more fiber, probiotics, flax or chia seed, and more water, among others, these did not help any of my problems. So, I just learned to live with the symptoms, and somehow, gave up searching for a solution. Those like me who suffer from a digestive condition know that it can be frustrating not understanding what food made us gassy or bloated and caused diarrhea or constipation and that constant fear that anything we eat can trigger the reactions.

The research for this book led me to plenty of new information and new approaches that gave me hope. I had not heard of the FODMAP diet before. But now, knowing how these foods can be problematic and cause an array of symptoms is relieving because I can work on determining which foods I need to eliminate. One of my problems, however, is that I love food! And following such a strict dietary approach seems like a monumental task. In my own way, though, I have eliminated or at least minimized the consumption of these foods and still trying to discover which foods mean trouble for me.

Because of my love for food, I had this bad habit of constantly snacking throughout the day and often not chewing my food properly. These bad behaviors, which I am now trying to change, probably worsened my situation.

Certainly, I also follow many of the tips I included in this book. I'm a fan of the Mediterranean diet and intermittent fasting. I stay physically active, go for walks and jogs, practice yoga and meditation, and include strength training exercises in my daily routines. In addition, I have tried many of the supplements and herbal remedies mentioned in Chapter 9. Multivitamins, vitamin D, and vitamin C are part of my daily use. I take supplements like probiotics, prebiotics, and digestive enzymes regularly; I may take a break and then retake them at another time. Do I feel they help all the time? Not always, but I think it's a good idea to take them when we feel we would really benefit from them. Similarly, there are others that I take on occasion, like oregano oil, MCT (coconut oil), or black seed oil.

As part of my research, I took an "intelligence" test, hoping it would help me identify the causes of my digestive problems. This test requires blood, stool, and saliva samples and is supposed to provide insights into the microbiome and other areas of our health. The results were mostly "Good" and "Not Optimal," especially in gas production like methane, which is often related to a SIBO condition where constipation is predominant. The company recommended their customized supplements to address the non-optimal conditions, and they provided lists of foods to avoid (for six months), foods to minimize, foods to enjoy, and a list of superfoods. Of course, the list of foods to avoid included high FODMAPs like mangoes, pistachios, broccoli, cauliflower, and asparagus, but it also had foods that I never eat, like caviar? And foods that are often considered healthy, like lemons and turmeric! Despite following their advice on taking their supplements and following these food lists, I can't tell yet whether that has made a huge difference in my digestive symptoms, mainly with bloating, which I regularly experience, regardless of what I eat. I feel, however, that troubles with gas and constipation have lessened a bit.

Despite not having found the perfect way to eat or the key supplement that will make my symptoms go away completely, I feel empowered now with the knowledge I've gained with this experience about how our bodies work, especially the connection of our gut and brain, how foods affect us, the benefits other supplements can provide, and healthy habits that are an important addition to our approach to manage our condition. I feel more aware and listen to the signs my body sends out. I feel confident I can make better choices that will be beneficial for my digestion and overall health. I keep in mind that, like everything in life, balance is essential; it isn't about avoiding this or that food or following this or that approach, but practicing everything in moderation.

I thank you again for reading Understanding Women's Gut Health. I sincerely hope you found it insightful, entertaining, and valuable in your journey. I would greatly appreciate it if you could take a moment to share your thoughts and **leave a review on Amazon.**

Just scan the QR code below!

Your feedback is incredibly important to me and helps other readers discover the book. Whether you loved it, found it helpful, or have constructive criticism to offer, your review will make a significant difference as it can help me reach more readers and continue creating content that resonates with you.

Leaving a review is simple:

- Visit the book's Amazon page.
- Scroll down to the "Customer Reviews" section.
- Click the "Write a customer review" button.

Thank you once again for choosing Understanding Women's Gut Health. I truly appreciate your support and look forward to hearing your thoughts.

Warm regards,
Julia Moreno

REFERENCES

About Olive Oil. "Does Olive Oil Lose Its Health Benefits When Heated?" https://www.aboutoliveoil.org/does-olive-oil-lose-its-health-benefits-when-heated. 07/25/2023

Akimbekov, Nuraly S., et al. "Vitamin D and the Host-Gut Microbiome: A Brief Overview." Acta Histochemica et Cytochemica, vol. 53, no. 3, 26 June 2020, pp. 33–42, www.ncbi.nlm.nih.gov/pmc/articles/PMC7322162/,

Alexander, James L., et al. "Gut Microbiota Modulation of Chemotherapy Efficacy and Toxicity." Nature Reviews Gastroenterology & Hepatology, vol. 14, no. 6, 8 Mar. 2017, pp. 356–365, www.nature.com/articles/nrgastro.2017.20,

Allan, S. A. (2022, July 20). "What is Leaky Gut Syndrome? Canadian Digestive Health Foundation." Retrieved November 30, 2022, from https://cdhf.ca/en/what-is-leaky-gut-syndrome/

Allert, Stefanie, et al. "Candida Albicans-Induced Epithelial Damage Mediates Translocation through Intestinal Barriers." MBio, vol. 9, no. 3, 2018, pp. e00915-, www.ncbi.nlm.nih.gov/pubmed/29871918.

"Aloe Information | Mount Sinai - New York." Mount Sinai Health System, www.mountsinai.org/health-library/herb/aloe. 07/25/23

Ang, Q. Y., et all. (2020). Ketogenic diets alter the gut microbiome resulting in decreased intestinal Th17 cells. Cell, 181(6), 1263-1275. https://doi.org/10.1016/j.cell.2020.04.027

Antunes, F, et al. "Autophagy and Intermittent Fasting: The Connection for Cancer Therapy?" Clinics, vol. 73, no. Suppl 1, 1 Dec. 2018, www.scielo.br/pdf/clin/v73s1/1807-5932-clin-73-e814s.pdf

Authier, Hélène, et al. "Synergistic Effects of Licorice Root and Walnut Leaf Extracts on Gastrointestinal Candidiasis, Inflammation and Gut Microbiota Composition in Mice." Microbiology Spectrum, vol. 10, no. 2, 27 Apr. 2022, p. e0235521, pubmed.ncbi.nlm.nih.gov/35262409/, https://doi.org/10.1128/spectrum.02355-21.

Baker, J. M., et al. (2017). "Estrogen–gut microbiome axis: physiological and clinical implications." Maturitas, 103, 45-53. www.ncbi.nlm.nih.gov/pubmed/28778332.

"Best Probiotics for Irritable Bowel Syndrome (IBS) Explained." Diet vs Disease, 11 May 2017, www.dietvsdisease.org/probiotics-ibs/.

BLACK SEED: Overview, Uses, Side Effects, Precautions, Interactions, Dosing and Reviews. (n.d.). https://www.webmd.com/vitamins/ai/ingredientmono-901/black-seed

Carabotti, Marilia, et al. "The Gut-Brain Axis: Interactions between Enteric Microbiota, Central and Enteric Nervous Systems." Annals of Gastroenterology, vol. 28, no. 2, 2015, pp. 203–209. https://www.ncbi.nlm.nih.gov/pmc/articles/PMC4367209/

Carnauba, Renata, et al. "Diet-Induced Low-Grade Metabolic Acidosis and Clinical Outcomes: A Review." Nutrients, vol. 9, no. 6, 25 May 2017, p. 538, https://doi.org/10.3390/nu9060538.

Celiac Disease and Women's Health | BeyondCeliac.org. (n.d.). Beyond Celiac. Retrieved November 30, 2022, from https://www.beyondceliac.org/living-with-celiac-disease/womens-health/

Chen, Li-Ru, et al. "Utilization of Isoflavones in Soybeans for Women with Menopausal Syndrome: An Overview." International Journal of Molecular Sciences, vol. 22, no. 6, 22 Mar. 2021, p. 3212, https://doi.org/10.3390/ijms22063212

Choung, Rok Seon, et al. "Irritable Bowel Syndrome and Chronic Pelvic Pain." Journal of Clinical Gastroenterology, Mar. 2010, p. 1, https://doi.org/10.1097/mcg.0b013e3181d7a368

Cleveland Clinic. "IBD, Ulcerative Colitis, Crohn's Disease, Symptoms, Treatment." Cleveland Clinic, 5 Mar. 2021, https://my.clevelandclinic.org/health/diseases/15587-inflammatory-bowel-disease-overview

Cleveland clinic. "Mediterranean Diet." Cleveland Clinic, 20 Nov. 2022, https://my.clevelandclinic.org/health/articles/16037-mediterranean-diet

Cognitive Behavioral Therapy for IBS. (2021, September). About IBS. Retrieved March 5, 2023, from https://aboutibs.org/treatment/psychological-treatments/cognitive-behavioral-therapy/

Costantini, Lara, et al. "Impact of Omega-3 Fatty Acids on the Gut Microbiota." International Journal of Molecular Sciences, vol. 18, no. 12, 2017, p. 2645, www.ncbi.nlm.nih.gov/pubmed/29215589, https://doi.org/10.3390/ijms18122645.

Diamanti-Kandarakis, et al. (2009). Insulin resistance in PCOS. Diagnosis and management of polycystic ovary syndrome, 35-61. https://pubmed.ncbi.nlm.nih.gov/23065822/

Didari, Tina, et al. "Effectiveness of Probiotics in Irritable Bowel Syndrome: Updated Systematic Review with Meta-Analysis." World Journal of Gastroenterology, vol. 21, no. 10, 2015, pp. 3072–84, www.ncbi.nlm.nih.gov/pubmed/25780308.

"Does Soy Cause Cancer?" Moffitt Cancer Center, 1 June 2021, www.moffitt.org/taking-care-of-your-health/taking-care-of-your-health-story-archive/does-soy-cause-cancer/. Accessed 24 July 2023.

Dukowicz, Andrew C., et al. "Small Intestinal Bacterial Overgrowth." Gastroenterology & Hepatology, vol. 3, no. 2, 1 Feb. 2007, pp. 112–122, www.ncbi.nlm.nih.gov/pmc/articles/PMC3099351/.

Edwards, Sara M., et al. "The Maternal Gut Microbiome during Pregnancy." MCN, the American Journal of Maternal/Child Nursing, Aug. 2017, p. 1, https://doi.org/10.1097/nmc.0000000000000372.

Elsenbruch, S. "Melatonin: A Novel Treatment for IBS?" Gut, vol. 54, no. 10, 1 Oct. 2005, pp. 1353–1354, https://doi.org/10.1136/gut.2005.074377.

"Five Natural Lectin Blockers Assist Your Gut Health (2023 Updated)." Healthcanal.com, 6 Feb. 2023, www.healthcanal.com/nutrition/lectin-blocker. Accessed 26 July 2023

FODMAP food list | Monash FODMAP - Monash Fodmap. 2019. https://www.monashfodmap.com/about-fodmap-and-ibs/high-and-low-fodmap-foods/

Gastroesophageal reflux disease (GERD) - Symptoms and causes. (2022, July 26). Mayo Clinic. Retrieved November 30, 2022, from https://www.mayoclinic.org/diseases-conditions/gerd/symptoms-causes/syc-20361940

Gearry, Richard, et al. "Efficacy of the Low FODMAP Diet for Treating Irritable Bowel Syndrome: The Evidence to Date." Clinical and Experimental Gastroenterology, vol. 9, June 2016, p. 131, www.ncbi.nlm.nih.gov/pmc/articles/PMC4918736/.

Genoni, Angela, et al. "Long-Term Paleolithic Diet Is Associated with Lower Resistant Starch Intake, Different Gut Microbiota Composition and Increased Serum TMAO Concentrations." European Journal of Nutrition, vol. 59, no. 5, 5 July 2019, pp. 1845–1858, https://doi.org/10.1007/s00394-019-02036-y.

Gigante, Isabella, et al. "Cannabinoid Receptors Overexpression in a Rat Model of Irritable Bowel Syndrome (IBS) after Treatment with a Ketogenic Diet." International Journal of Molecular Sciences, vol. 22, no. 6, 1 Jan. 2021, p. 2880, www.mdpi.com/1422-0067/22/6/2880/htm

Günther, Claudia, et al. "The Gut-Brain Axis in Inflammatory Bowel Disease—Current and Future Perspectives." International Journal of Molecular

Sciences, vol. 22, no. 16, 18 Aug. 2021, p. 8870, www.ncbi.nlm.nih.gov/pmc/articles/PMC8396333/.

Guo, Shanshan, et al. "Ginger Alleviates DSS-Induced Ulcerative Colitis Severity by Improving the Diversity and Function of Gut Microbiota." Frontiers in Pharmacology, vol. 12, 22 Feb. 2021, https://doi.org/10.3389/fphar.2021.632569.

How nightshades affect arthritis | Arthritis Foundation. (n.d.). https://www.arthritis.org/health-wellness/healthy-living/nutrition/anti-inflammatory/how-nightshades-affect-arthritis. Accessed 25 July 2023

"Hypnosis for IBS." IFFGD-International Foundation for Gastrointestinal Disorders, https://aboutibs.org/treatment/complimentary-or-alternative-treatments/hypnosis-for-ibs/. Accessed 24 July 2023.

IBS Diet: What to Do and What to Avoid - about IBS. 8 Mar. 2021, https://aboutibs.org/treatment/ibs-diet/ibs-diet-what-to-do-and-what-to-avoid/#: Accessed 26 July 2023

Jia, Manyi, et al. "Effects of Medium Chain Fatty Acids on Intestinal Health of Monogastric Animals." Current Protein & Peptide Science, vol. 21, no. 8, pp. 777–784, 2020. https://benthamscience.com/article/103359

Jurenka, J. S. (2009). Anti-inflammatory properties of curcumin, a major constituent of Curcuma longa: a review of preclinical and clinical research. Alternative medicine review, 14(2). https://altmedrev.com/wp-content/uploads/2019/02/v14-2-141.pdf. 07/25/2023

Kavuri, Vijaya, et al. "Irritable Bowel Syndrome: Yoga as Remedial Therapy." Evidence-Based Complementary and Alternative Medicine, vol. 2015, 2015, pp. 1–10, https://doi.org/10.1155/2015/398156.

Kennedy, Paul J. "Irritable Bowel Syndrome: A Microbiome-Gut-Brain Axis Disorder?" World Journal of Gastroenterology, vol. 20, no. 39, 2014, p. 14105, https://doi.org/10.3748/wjg.v20.i39.14105

Khanijow, Vikesh, et al. "Sleep Dysfunction and Gastrointestinal Diseases." Gastroenterology & Hepatology, vol. 11, no. 12, 2015, pp. 817–25, www.ncbi.nlm.nih.gov/pmc/articles/PMC4849511

Kim, Young Sun, et al. "Sex-Gender Differences in Irritable Bowel Syndrome." Journal of Neurogastroenterology and Motility, vol. 24, no. 4, 1 Oct. 2018, pp. 544–558, www.jnmjournal.org/journal/view.html?uid=1423&vmd=Full&

Kirkpatrick, B., & Miller, B. J. (2013). Inflammation and schizophrenia. Schizophrenia Bulletin, 39(6), 1174–1179. https://doi.org/10.1093/schbul/sbt141

Kuo, Braden, et al. "Genomic and Clinical Effects Associated with a Relaxation Response Mind-Body Intervention in Patients with Irritable Bowel Syndrome and Inflammatory Bowel Disease." PLOS ONE, vol. 10, no. 4, 30 Apr. 2015, p. e0123861, https://doi.org/10.1371/journal.pone.0123861

"Lectins." The Nutrition Source, 24 Jan. 2019, www.hsph.harvard.edu/nutrition source/anti-nutrients/lectins/

Liu, Manman, et al. Apigenin Inhibits the Histamine-Induced Proliferation of Ovarian Cancer Cells by Downregulating ERα/ERβ Expression. Vol. 11, 8 Sept. 2021, https://www.ncbi.nlm.nih.gov/pmc/articles/PMC8456091/.

LiverTox: Clinical and Research Information on Drug-Induced Liver Injury [Internet]. Bethesda (MD): National Institute of Diabetes and Digestive and Kidney Diseases; 2012-. Oregano. [Updated 2023 Apr 28]. https://www.ncbi.nlm.nih.gov/books/NBK591556/

Lozupone, Catherine A, et al. "Diversity, stability and resilience of the human gut microbiota." Nature. 2012 Sep 13;489(7415):220-30. www.ncbi.nlm.nih.gov/pmc/articles/PMC3577372/

Marteau, Philippe, et al. "Tolerance of Probiotics and Prebiotics." Journal of Clinical Gastroenterology, vol. 38, no. Supplement 2, July 2004, pp. S67–S69, https://doi.org/10.1097/01.mcg.0000128929.37156.a7.

Mastromarino, Paola, et all. M. E. (2014). Correlation between lactoferrin and beneficial microbiota in breast milk and infant's feces. Biometals, 27(5), 1077-1086. d.docksci.com/correlation-between-lactoferrin-and-beneficial-microbiota-in-breast-milk-and-inf_5ad0894cd64ab22af2958b5d.html

Mayo Clinic Staff. "Meditation: A Simple, Fast Way to Reduce Stress." Mayo Clinic, 22 Apr. 2020, www.mayoclinic.org/tests-procedures/meditation/in-depth/meditation/art-20045858

Mentella, Maria Chiara, et al. "Cancer and Mediterranean Diet: A Review." Nutrients, vol. 11, no. 9, 2 Sept. 2019, p. 2059, www.ncbi.nlm.nih.gov/pmc/articles/PMC6770822/.

Mlcek, Jiri, et al. "Quercetin and Its Anti-Allergic Immune Response." Molecules, vol. 21, no. 5, 12 May 2016, p. 623, www.ncbi.nlm.nih.gov/pmc/articles/PMC6273625/

Mulak, A., Taché, et al. (2014). Sex hormones in the modulation of irritable bowel syndrome. World journal of gastroenterology: WJG, 20(10), 2433. www.wjgnet.com/1007-9327/full/v20/i10/2433.htm , https://doi.org/10.3748/wjg.v20.i10.2433

Nagpal, Ravinder, et al. "Gut Microbiome-Mediterranean Diet Interactions in

Improving Host Health." F1000Research, vol. 8, 21 May 2019, p. 699, https://doi.org/10.12688/f1000research.18992.1

Neroni, Bruna, et al. "Relationship between Sleep Disorders and Gut Dysbiosis: What Affects What?" Sleep Medicine, vol. 87, 1 Nov. 2021, pp. 1–7, www.sciencedirect.com/science/article/pii/S1389945721004354?via%3Dihub, https://doi.org/10.1016/j.sleep.2021.08.003.

Nielsen, Elsa Sandberg, et al. "Lacto-Fermented Sauerkraut Improves Symptoms in IBS Patients Independent of Product Pasteurisation – a Pilot Study." Food & Function, vol. 9, no. 10, 17 Oct. 2018, pp. 5323–5335, https://pubs.rsc.org/en/content/articlelanding/2018/fo/c8fo00968f/unauth#

Qiu, Peng, et al. "The Gut Microbiota in Inflammatory Bowel Disease." Frontiers in Cellular and Infection Microbiology, vol. 12, 22 Feb. 2022, https://doi.org/10.3389/fcimb.2022.733992.

Ratajczak, Alicja Ewa, et al. "Vitamin c Deficiency and the Risk of Osteoporosis in Patients with an Inflammatory Bowel Disease." Nutrients, vol. 12, no. 8, 1 Aug. 2020, p. 2263, www.mdpi.com/2072-6643/12/8/2263/htm, https://doi.org/10.3390/nu12082263.

Rinninella, Emanuele, et al. "What Is the Healthy Gut Microbiota Composition? A Changing Ecosystem across Age, Environment, Diet, and Diseases." Microorganisms, vol. 7, no. 1, 10 Jan. 2019, p. 14, www.ncbi.nlm.nih.gov/pmc/articles/PMC6351938/, https://doi.org/10.3390/microorganisms7010014.

Sansone, Randy A., et al. "IRRITABLE BOWEL SYNDROME: Relationships with Abuse in Childhood." Innovations in Clinical Neuroscience, vol. 12, no. 5-6, 2015, pp. 34–37, www.ncbi.nlm.nih.gov/pmc/articles/PMC4479362/

SCL Health. (2018). Oil Essentials: The 5 Healthiest Cooking Oils. Retrieved February 28, 2023, from https://www.sclhealth.org/blog/2021/05/oil-essentials-the-5-healthiest-cooking-oils/

Shahabi, Leila, et al. "Self-Regulation Evaluation of Therapeutic Yoga and Walking for Patients with Irritable Bowel Syndrome: A Pilot Study." Psychology, Health & Medicine, vol. 21, no. 2, 18 June 2015, pp. 176–188, https://doi.org/10.1080/13548506.2015.1051557.

Sharma, Dave Krishan, et al. "Augmented Glutathione Absorption from Oral Mucosa and Its Effect on Skin Pigmentation: A Clinical Review." Clinical, Cosmetic and Investigational Dermatology, vol. Volume 15, Sept. 2022, pp. 1853–1862, https://doi.org/10.2147/ccid.s378470.

"Slippery Elm". (n.d.). Mount Sinai Health System. /https://www.mountsinai.org/health-library/herb/slippery-elm. 07/25/2023

Soulaidopoulos, Stergios, et al. "Overview of Chios Mastic Gum (Pistacia Lentiscus) Effects on Human Health." Nutrients, vol. 14, no. 3, 28 Jan. 2022, p. 590, https://doi.org/10.3390/nu14030590.

Su, Junhong, et al. "Remodeling of the Gut Microbiome during Ramadan-Associated Intermittent Fasting." The American Journal of Clinical Nutrition, vol. 113, no. 5, 12 Apr. 2021, pp. 1332–1342, https://doi.org/10.1093/ajcn/nqaa388.

Sugaya, Nagisa, et al. "Effect of Prolonged Stress on the Adrenal Hormones of Individuals with Irritable Bowel Syndrome." BioPsychoSocial Medicine, vol. 9, no. 1, 23 Jan. 2015, https://doi.org/10.1186/s13030-015-0031-7

Sun, Li-Juan, et al. "Gut Hormones in Microbiota-Gut-Brain Cross-Talk." Chinese Medical Journal, vol. 133, no. 7, Apr. 2020, pp. 826–833, https://doi.org/10.1097/cm9.0000000000000706.   https://mednexus.org/doi/full/10.1097/CM9.0000000000000706

"The Benefits of Intermittent Fasting for Sleep." Sleep Foundation, 3 June 2021, www.sleepfoundation.org/physical-health/intermittent-fasting-sleep#:~

Thompson, Robert S., et al. "Dietary Prebiotics and Bioactive Milk Fractions Improve NREM Sleep, Enhance REM Sleep Rebound and Attenuate the Stress-Induced Decrease in Diurnal Temperature and Gut Microbial Alpha Diversity." Frontiers in Behavioral Neuroscience, vol. 10, 10 Jan. 2017, https://doi.org/10.3389/fnbeh.2016.00240.

Tomova, Aleksandra, et al. "The Effects of Vegetarian and Vegan Diets on Gut Microbiota." Frontiers in Nutrition, vol. 6, no. 47, 17 Apr. 2019, https://doi.org/10.3389/fnut.2019.00047.

Unal, Mehmet, et al. "Evaluation of Frequency of Irritable Bowel Syndrome in Patients with Chronic Urticaria." Journal of Turgut Ozal Medical Center, 2018, p. 1, https://doi.org/10.5455/jtomc.2018.02.026.

"Unique Gut Microbiome Patterns Linked to Healthy Aging, Increased Longevity." May 13, 2021, 13 May 2021, www.nia.nih.gov/news/unique-gut-microbiome-patterns-linked-healthy-aging-increased-longevity . Accessed 23 July 2023.

University of California - Los Angeles. (2019, September 6). Study shows how serotonin and a popular anti-depressant affect the gut's microbiota. https://www.sciencedaily.com/releases/2019/09/190906092809.htm

Villines, Z. (2021b, April 28). "What natural remedies are there for Crohn's disease?" https://www.medicalnewstoday.com/articles/natural-remedies-for-crohns.

Wang, Yanan, et al. "Sleep and the Gut Microbiota in Preschool-Aged Children." *Sleep*, vol. 45, no. 6, 17 Jan. 2022, https://pubmed.ncbi.nlm.nih.gov/35037059/.

WebMD Editorial Contributors. "Health Benefits of Fennel." WebMD, WebMD, 11 Sept. 2020, www.webmd.com/food-recipes/health-benefits-fennel%23:~07/25/2023

"What Impact Does the Keto Diet Have on Gut Microbiome & Long Term Health?" Center for Nutrition Studies, 13 Feb. 2020, https://nutritionstudies.org/what-impact-does-the-keto-diet-have-on-gut-microbiome-long-term-health/

Wheless, James W. "History of the Ketogenic Diet." Epilepsia, vol. 49 Suppl 8, no. s8, 4 Nov. 2008, pp. 3–5, www.ncbi.nlm.nih.gov/pubmed/19049574

Women and Irritable Bowel Syndrome (IBS). Faculty and Investigators at the UNC Center for Functional GI & Motility Disorders Conducted a National Survey of the Effects of Changes in Female Sex Hormones on Irritable Bowel Symptoms. https://www.med.unc.edu/ibs/wp-content/uploads/sites/450/2017/10/IBS-in-Women.pdf

"World-First Study Shows Benefits of 5:2 Diet for People with Diabetes." *Home*, https://unisa.edu.au/Media-Centre/Releases/2018/World-first-study-shows-benefits-of-52-diet-for-people-with-diabetes.

Yan, Li-hui, et al. "Association between Small Intestinal Bacterial Overgrowth and Beta-Cell Function of Type 2 Diabetes." Journal of International Medical Research, vol. 48, no. 7, July 2020, p. 030006052093786, https://doi.org/10.1177/0300060520937866

Yang, T., Chen, C., Lin, C., Lin, W., Kuo, C., & Kao, C. (2015). Risk for irritable bowel syndrome in fibromyalgia patients. Medicine, 94(10), e616. https://doi.org/10.1097/md.0000000000000616

Zhang, Husen, et al. "Host Adaptive Immunity Alters Gut Microbiota." The ISME Journal, vol. 9, no. 3, 12 Sept. 2014, pp. 770–781, https://doi.org/10.1038/ismej.2014.165

Made in the USA
Monee, IL
14 November 2024

70153538R00098